WHAT YOU DON'T KNOW MAY HURT YOU—AND YOUR BABY

Whether you are already pregnant or just deciding it's time to have a child, you need to ask important questions about everything that influences your health and the health of your baby. You might wonder if any over-the-counter drugs can cause birth defects. If airplane travel poses a risk. Whether you should exercise—and how much. What medical tests are necessary, and which carry hidden dangers. Or you might want to know more about food additives and special diets. Now you can find the answers to all your questions in this vital reference work that's easy to understand, sensitively written, and packed with up-to-date, scientifically sound information. You can't afford to be without it.

The Safe Pregnancy Book

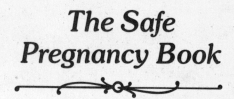

CAROL ANN RINZLER is a medical writer whose other books include: *The Children's Medicine Chest; The Consumer's Guide to Household Products; Cosmetics: What the Ads Don't Tell You; The Dictionary of Medical Folklore; The Signet Book of Chocolate; The Signet Book of Yogurt;* and *Strictly Female,* available in a Plume edition. She is a columnist for *American Health* magazine.

The Safe Pregnancy Book

by

Carol Ann Rinzler

Foreword by Niels H. Lauersen, M.D.

A PLUME BOOK

NEW AMERICAN LIBRARY

NEW YORK AND SCARBOROUGH, ONTARIO

Copyright © 1984 by Carol Ann Rinzler

Foreword copyright © 1984 by New American Library

PLUME TRADEMARK REG. U.S. PAT. OFF. AND FOREIGN COUNTRIES
REG. TRADEMARK—MARCA REGISTRADA
HECHO EN HARRISONBURG, VA., U.S.A.

SIGNET, SIGNET CLASSIC, MENTOR, PLUME, MERIDIAN
and NAL BOOKS
are published *in the United States* by New American Library,
1633 Broadway, New York, New York 10019
in Canada by The New American Library of Canada Limited,
81 Mack Avenue, Scarborough, Ontario M1L 1M8

LIBRARY OF CONGRESS CATALOGING IN PUBLICATION DATA

Rinzler, Carol Ann.
  The safe pregnancy book.

  Bibliography
  Includes index.
  1. Pregnancy. 2. Obstetrics—Popular works.
I. Title.
RG525.R54   1985   618.2′4   84-20571
ISBN 0-452-25610-0

First Printing, January, 1985

2 3 4 5 6 7 8 9

PRINTED IN THE UNITED STATES OF AMERICA

For
Jacqueline K. Barton
and
Klaus G. Grohmann,
RIGOROUS SCHOLARS,
IMAGINATIVE TEACHERS,
WHO OPENED THE WAY
TO A WORLD FULL OF WONDERS

ACKNOWLEDGMENTS

I am indebted to a number of people whose generous assistance helped to make this book a reality. Among them are Nikki Field, who added a note of practical experience to my research; Wendy Chavkin, M.D., Connie Miller, M.D., Donald Pizzarello, M.D., Pedro Rosso, M.D., Jeanne Stellman, Ph.D., and Marcia Storch, M.D., each of whom was kind enough to read and comment upon a portion of the manuscript; and Carole Hall and Phyllis Westberg, whose clear thought and reasoned criticism helped to make everything work.

Contents

PART III   Drugs

PART IV   Medical Procedures

PART V   Nutrition

PART VI   The Environment

PART VII   Tests You Should Know About

A Note to The Reader

When talking about pregnancy and childbirth, it is well to remember that safety is relative. As in other situations in life, there is no absolutely safe course to follow; there are only those that may reduce—or increase—the relative risk involved.

The material in this book, drawn from research current at the time the book was written, is presented for your information only. None of it should be regarded as a prescription for a risk-free pregnancy, nor should any of the information here be substituted for your own doctor's advice or adopted without his or her consent. Your doctor is the person most familiar with your own medical history and current state of health. Therefore, he or she is the person best qualified to offer medical advice when you want to become pregnant, while you are pregnant, when you are ready to deliver your baby and while you are nursing.

Please note that the adverse effects attributed to some of the substances, devices and procedures described here may not happen to every person who uses them or every time the substances, devices and procedures are used. Once again, therefore, your own doctor is your best guide to the effect they may have on you or your partner.

Finally, please note that some of the product names used in this book are registered trademarks.

Foreword

Most of today's modern, educated women are carefully planning their families. The babies I help to deliver into this world are more likely to be one of two, rather than one of four, offspring. Many times a newborn I cradle in my hands will remain an "only child." I hear the reasons why from my own patients. Facing practical issues, such as their own life goals and the high cost of raising a daughter or a son, women and men wait until the "right time" to conceive. This approach means families are smaller than they were generations ago, but on the other hand, each child has the chance to be more profoundly cherished.

In this time of planned motherhood, women have become particularly health-conscious. They want the children they are creating to be as robust as nature will allow. Conscientiously, they study the ways that they can successfully conceive and carry a baby to term. Never, to my knowledge, have women known more about their bodies than they do right now. Yet there is always more to discover.

In their search for awareness, expectant mothers and women who want to become pregnant will find that *The Safe Pregnancy Book* will protectively guide them through the transition into parenthood. Today's women are facing more options than their mothers did. Choices among medications, vitamins, foods that may be chemically treated must be made. The use of alcohol, tobacco, caffeine has to be controlled. Generations ago I'm sure that women tried to stay healthy and eat well, but they didn't know what science has only recently taught us.

Medical researchers have learned more about substances, such as drugs, that might affect a developing fetus than they did in the past. However, this knowledge has meant greater responsibility for the expectant mother. Now, along with her personal health habits, she has environmental health hazards to consider. For instance, if she enters a newly painted room, there may be toxic elements in the paint that, once inhaled, might cross the placenta and touch her unborn child. Products that might not harm a grown woman may be unsafe for the infant in her womb.

Every woman wants to understand the best steps to take for a healthy conception and pregnancy. Not a day goes by that a pregnant, or trying-to-be pregnant, woman doesn't call and ask about a medication she questions, or a food additive she has noticed in something she has eaten, or an activity she thinks may have stressed her reproductive system. These queries led me to write *Childbirth with Love,* and to recommend with conviction *The Safe Pregnancy Book.*

This volume can be with you from the moment you decide that you'd like to be a mother, until the time you are comforting and nursing your baby. Carol Ann Rinzler clears up many uncertainties: issues like airplane travel, the effect of exercise on pregnancy, the safety of medical tests, prescription and nonprescription drugs— these are just a few of her subjects.

If you are holding this book in your hands, the odds are that you're pregnant or thinking about conceiving. With this easy-to-use reference I believe you've found a way to make nine expectant months a safer passage for you and your baby.

—Niels H. Lauersen, M.D.

Introduction

Are you pregnant now?

Do you hope to be soon?

Then there's a good chance that you've wondered whether your baby will be normal; every prospective parent does.

It is a happy fact of life that the vast majority of pregnancies— 92 to 96 percent or more—will end beautifully with the birth of a healthy baby. But there's no denying the fact that some children will be born with problems and that you have every right to be concerned. It's a natural expression of your love and sense of responsibility for your baby-to-be.

Our grandmothers relied on aphorisms ("Eating strawberries while you are pregnant will 'mark' the baby") and old wives' tales to ease their uncertainty, but our understanding of how birth defects occur has taken us far beyond folklore. Today we know that what we eat or drink or how we live or where we work may affect our unborn children, and we are careful to consider what we do while we are pregnant or trying to conceive.

For example: The truly successful conception is one in which an intact, healthy sperm meets an intact, healthy egg to create a new organism with the best chance of implanting in the uterus and thriving through the nine months of pregnancy. So, when you are trying to conceive, you will be concerned with the things that might interfere with the ability to produce and deliver the healthy sperm and egg, functions so commonplace that we often take them for granted, forgetting for the moment how wonderfully miraculous they really are.

While you are pregnant, you and your baby are essentially one person. You share the same environment, and virtually everything to which you are exposed will eventually affect him, one way or another. You need to know which foods, drugs, chemicals and other things in your life may harm your child or affect your natural ability to carry him successfully to term.

Whether you choose to have your baby at home, or in a birthing center, or in a hospital, there is likely to come a time when your energies are so taken up with the physical business of labor and birth that you will have to trust someone else to make important medical decisions for you both. As delivery comes closer, you will certainly be concerned with the drugs and procedures that may affect your baby during childbirth, and the relationship between you and your doctor or midwife will be very important.

After the long months of pregnancy, when you and your baby become entirely separate people, your decision to nurse can provide a connection rich in physical and emotional rewards for both of you. Your immediate concern will be with the foods, drugs and other aspects of your health or life-style that might affect your ability to produce the nutritious milk your baby needs.

This book aims to provide information that can ease or illuminate these concerns at each stage of childbearing. How best to use what you find here? Rely on your own natural good sense:

1. Read carefully, and don't panic. To keep a sense of balance, you need to remember to look for the qualifiers—words like "may" and "perhaps." Because it can take years to prove or invalidate a new theory, researchers are likely to be very cautious about drawing absolute conclusions, and you should be, too.

2. Be realistic about risk factors. There's a big difference between being intelligently aware of the risks you and your baby may face during pregnancy and scaring yourself silly about things you will never encounter. It's true, for example, that many drugs, chemicals and medical conditions can play havoc with your reproductive system or damage a developing fetus—but only if you are exposed to them. As a rule of thumb, though not an absolute one, you can assume that the more exotic the risk is, the less likely you are to run into it. Major genetic disorders, for example, affect only a relatively small group of people, while cigarette smoking, which seems so prosaic, is pervasive in our society. Statistically speaking, your baby is far more likely to be damaged by cigarette smoking (yours or your partner's) than by an esoteric genetic disorder or industrial chemical hazard. It does bear thinking about, doesn't it?

3. Moderate your behavior to protect your baby. When you are pregnant or want to be, don't smoke. Don't use illicit drugs. Eat well. See your doctor regularly, both for preconception counseling and for prenatal care. These simple guidelines can pay immeasurable dividends in safety for your baby at a time when you are, sentimentally and realistically, "living for two." And by the way, babies have mothers *and* fathers: these guidelines apply to both of you.

4. Pick a doctor whose judgment you trust. No matter how independent you are, how intelligent or how in charge of your own life, there may come a time when you will have to trust your doctor to make a medical decision for you. That's got nothing to do with your intelligence or your independence; it's just a practical fact of life. That's why you need to look hard for someone you respect.

Remember that science moves swiftly. Some of the research reported in this book, though current as I write, may have been invalidated by the time you get to read it. Check with your doctor, who is most familiar with your medical history, before deciding that anything reported here applies to you.

C.R.

Part I

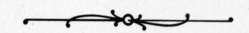

Personal Health

1. How Old Are You?

Psychologically, people who wait until they are in their late twenties or thirties or even their forties before having a baby have a number of things in their favor. Because they are older, they may have a surer sense of how they want to live their lives and raise their children. Their economic situation is likely to be more secure, and they are probably able to deal more realistically with the physical problems that may arise during pregnancy.

On the other hand, waiting until you are older may make it more difficult to conceive or to carry a healthy baby to term.

How Age Affects Fertility

It is easiest for a woman to conceive when she is in her late teens or early twenties, for fertility seems to decline as women grow older.

One reason this happens is that our bodies are changing. Older women are more likely than young ones to have physiological problems that interfere with conception. They may have endometriosis (a proliferation of the tissue that lines the uterus), or they may have fibroid tumors. The first can block the fallopian tubes, preventing sperm and egg from meeting. The second may keep a fertilized egg from implanting successfully in the wall of the uterus.

Older women are also more likely to give birth to a child with Down's syndrome. The risk of producing a baby with Down's syndrome resulting from an extra chromosome (a condition known as trisomy 21) begins to rise when a woman is in her middle thirties. Between the ages of 35 and 39, the chances of having such a baby are between 1/500 and 1/200; between the ages of 40 to 45, the risk has risen to 2/200–6/200.

Nobody knows exactly why this should be so, but there are a few possible explanations. One is that the eggs in a woman's ovaries, formed before she herself was born, may degenerate as she grows older. Or, it may be that older couples have intercourse less frequently. This means that the sperm (which can live for several days in a woman's reproductive tract) may not be fresh when they meet a mature egg, or, conversely, sperm may not meet egg until the egg has traveled all the way down the fallopian tube, aging as it goes. Either way, the meeting—called delayed fertilization—is thought to be linked to an increased risk of chromosomal abnormalities in the fetus.

How Age Affects Pregnancy

There is a lot of research showing that women who become pregnant when they are very young (in their early teens) or quite a bit older (in their late thirties or forties) are more likely than other women to have problems, but whether the culprit is their age or a lack of good, solid prenatal care is still an open question.

Girls who get pregnant while still in their middle or early teens are much more likely than older mothers to develop anemia or toxemia or to deliver premature or low-birthweight babies. To some extent, this may be due simply to the physical immaturity of their bodies, but it's also possible that the connection may be socioeconomic, not physical. In other words, when girls are taught how to eat well during pregnancy and are cared for in the months before they give birth, the rate of complications during pregnancy may fall.

Older women are more likely to have problems delivering a normal flow of oxygen to the fetus. There's nothing mysterious about this: it's just the result of the normal aging and narrowing of the blood vessels, including those that supply the uterus. On the other hand, if an older woman's blood vessels are in good shape and she is healthy, good prenatal care can go a long way toward making her pregnancy successful. While this does not mean that good prenatal care can eliminate every complication that may arise during labor and delivery, many obstetricians suggest that how long you labor and how difficult your delivery is may depend more on the kind of prenatal care you got than on your age.

Having Your First Baby:
How Your Age Affects Your Chances of Carrying Safely to Term

Age of mother	Fetal deaths per 1,000 births
All women	5.3
30–34 years	5.8
Over 34 years	10

Source: National Center for Health Statistics.

Age holds fewer proven risks for fathers-to-be. Although the level of testosterone (male hormone) in a man's body may decline as he grows older, there doesn't seem to be any corresponding decline in sperm production. A potent man may be fertile at any age.

There is very little information about whether or not older fathers are more likely than young ones to produce babies with specific birth defects, although the incidence of Down's syndrome is now known to rise with the father's age, regardless of how old the mother is. To some extent, this certainly represents the medical community's focusing on the mother as the only parent involved in a pregnancy. But it's also important to point out that unlike a woman's eggs, which were produced before she was born and age along with her, sperm are being produced all the time. Every one is a fresh, new cell.

2. How Much Do You Weigh?

So long as he is neither emaciated nor starving (starvation causes the testes to shrink), how much a man weighs doesn't seem to have any bearing at all on his ability to produce normal amounts of healthy sperm.

For women, it's a different story. Being either very thin or very fat may interfere with a woman's ability to ovulate. Any sudden change in weight—even as little as five pounds up or down—can do the same thing. So can the starvation associated wtih anorexia nervosa or with even a more socially acceptable, long-term, very-low-calorie diet. Luckily, this kind of infertility is reversible; it usually disappears when a woman returns to her "normal" weight.

Being too fat or too thin can cause problems for a pregnant woman, too. Women who are very thin are more likely than other women to deliver a low-birthweight infant. Women who are very much overweight are more likely to develop hypertension that can affect the flow of blood to their fetus.

In labor, a very small woman (particularly a teenager) may have a difficult time because her pelvis is too small to accommodate a normal-size infant's head. A woman who is very much overweight may, because of her larger body size, require larger amounts of anesthesia, or she may hemorrhage more easily, or she may take longer to heal after childbirth.

3. Do You Have an Infectious Disease?

An infectious disease is any illness caused by a microorganism (bacteria, viruses, spirochetes, protozoas, or worms and their relatives). Infectious diseases may affect your fertility, damage a developing fetus or make labor and delivery more difficult for you or more dangerous for your baby.

Infections That May Make You Less Fertile

The fever that sometimes accompanies an infection may make a man temporarily less fertile by slowing or stopping the normal production of sperm. According to a report delivered to the American Occupational Health Conference in Los Angeles in 1984, a fever of 104°F or higher can produce temporary infertility that begins about a month after the fever and lasts for perhaps three months after that.

Mumps, which does not affect a child's reproductive system, can play havoc with an adult male's, causing atrophy of the testicles that leads to sterility even though hormone production stays unchanged.

A vaginal infection may change the acid/base balance (pH) of the vagina so that sperm have a hard time surviving there and thus cannot swim up to penetrate and fertilize a waiting egg.

Gonorrhea can impair fertility in both men and women. In women, gonorrhea is a "silent" disease that can scar and block the fallopian tubes without a woman's even knowing she has the infection. A mature egg cannot pass through the scarred tubes to meet the sperm. In men, gonorrhea may scar the epididymides, the tiny tubes through which the sperm must pass on their way out of the testicles; again, the result is that sperm and egg cannot meet.

Will Your Baby-to-Be Catch What You've Got?

Sometimes the organism that causes an infectious disease can cross the placenta and harm the fetus.

Chicken pox. There have been a few reports suggesting that if a woman catches chicken pox early in her pregnancy, between the ninth and the eleventh weeks, her baby may be born with skin lesions or physical defects. Later in pregnancy, chicken pox's ill effects on the fetus seem to be limited to skin lesions, although if a woman catches the infection in the last few days before she delivers, her baby may pick it up at birth.

Cytomegalovirus. This virus, also known as CMV, is similar to the virus that causes herpes infections. In adults, CMV infections may resemble mononucleosis or hepatitis or they may not cause any symptoms at all. When you are pregnant, though, a CMV infection can be very dangerous. The virus can cross the placenta and damage a growing fetus. Infants infected with CMV in the uterus may be aborted spontaneously, or they may die soon after birth, or they may be born alive with liver or blood disorders or an abnormally small head or weighing much less than they should. Some CMV-infected babies look perfectly normal at birth but develop hearing problems later on. There is no cure for CMV, which is spread by personal contact; cleanliness is the best line of defense.

Herpes. The herpes virus may (rarely) cross the placenta from mother to child. According to a 1984 report in the *Journal of the American Medical Association,* intrauterine herpes infections may account for up to 30 percent of all miscarriages. A baby who contracts herpes while still in the womb and survives may be born with an abnormally small head or with malformed eyes.

Hepatitis. The hepatitis virus crosses the placenta. Babies born to mothers who have the disease while they are pregnant may also be infected. In one study, 35 percent of the babies born with hepatitis were also low-birthweight. Some infants infected in the uterus are asymptomatic carriers. One fascinating 1978 study discovered that when either of a pair of parents tested positive for hepatitis antibodies, the babies they produced were more likely to be boys.

Mumps. While studies of human beings during the 1950s, 1960s and early in the 1970s failed to show any ill effects on the fetus when its mother had mumps while she was pregnant, later animal research has suggested the possibility that infants born to mothers infected with mumps may have a higher-than-normal incidence of heart defects.

Rubella. A rubella infection early in pregnancy is very likely to damage a developing fetus, causing mental retardation or physical defects. The likelihood of rubella's causing birth defects lessens later in pregnancy. (See *25. Testing for Rubella Antibodies.*)

Syphilis. Syphilis organisms cross the placenta and may cause a lot of different birth defects in a growing fetus. Babies born with congenital syphilis (syphilis acquired in the womb) may die soon after birth, or they may look healthy and normal but succumb later to an advanced form of the disease. If a pregnant woman with syphilis is treated before the fourth month of her pregnancy, the chances of her passing the disease on to her baby decline dramatically; treatment later in pregnancy does not seem to offer the same protection.

How Infectious Diseases Affect Labor and Delivery

According to a report presented at the 1984 annual meeting of the Society of Perinatal Obstetricians, women with nonspecific vaginitis (NSV), a vaginal infection not attributed to any specific organism, although it is thought to be caused by a bacterium, are two or three times more likely than other women to go into labor prematurely. NSV has also been associated with low-birthweight infants.

If you have chlamydia, gonorrhea, or an active case of genital herpes when you go into labor, your baby has a serious chance of picking up your infection as he travels down the birth canal.

In the newborn, chlamydia may cause a crusty form of eye

infection; gonorrhea may cause blindness; and herpes is a life-threatening infection. To protect your baby from the blindness caused by undetected gonorrhea, most states require the attending physician to put protective drops in her eyes as soon as she is born. However, the only sure way to protect a baby against these infections is a cesarean delivery which avoids the trip through the vaginal passageway. (See *29. Tests That Start after Labor Begins*.)

4. Do You Have a Chronic Condition or Long-Term Disability?

In most cases, a long-term illness or disability is less likely to interfere with your conceiving a baby than with your successfully carrying it to term. A notable exception, of course, would be any physical or neurological disorder that interferes with potency.

Bowel disease. According to a 1982 report delivered to the American Academy of Gastroenterologists, women who have active bowel disease (Crohn's disease, ulcerative colitis) while they are pregnant are more likely than other women to miscarry, go into labor prematurely or give birth to a baby with birth defects. Exactly why this should be so remains a mystery. It might seem logical to suspect that the sulfa drugs sometimes used to treat these conditions are the cause of the defects, but the fact is that the researchers who presented the 1982 report were unable to establish any cause-and-effect relationship between individual medications and specific defects.

Diabetes. Pregnancy complicates diabetes (the death rate for pregnant diabetics is twice that for other pregnant women), and diabetes complicates pregnancy. Women with diabetes are more likely to lose their babies before birth. In patients who have had diabetes for more than 10 years before becoming pregnant, the intrauterine fetal death rate approaches 20 percent; it doubles to 40 percent for women whose diabetes is complicated by damage to the blood vessels supplying the kidneys. Pregnant diabetics are more likely to deliver their babies stillborn; in fact, a history of unexplained stillbirths may be a warning sign of diabetes. Babies born live to diabetics are usually larger than other babies, but their size is deceptive because they are likely to be physically immature and must be regarded (from a medical standpoint) as premature. Finally, the risk of having a baby with congenital malformations is three times higher if you are a diabetic. Most birth defects in the babies of diabetic mothers occur very early in pregnancy, before the mother even knows she is pregnant and can adjust her medication to her new metabolic needs.

For all these reasons, many doctors warn against a diabetic woman's becoming pregnant more than twice, and some advise against any pregnancy at all. Obviously, individual cases require individual medical evaluation. For, despite all the potential problems, and despite the fact that managing a diabetic woman's pregnancy may represent a real challenge to the physician and patient alike, new methods of control mean that it may be possible for her to carry her pregnancy successfully to term. Women with diabetes may be advised to deliver by cesarean so as to spare both the mother and the child the stress of a prolonged labor.

Heart disease. Ordinarily, if a woman with heart disease becomes pregnant, her fetus may face two specific problems: (1) he may not be able to get all the oxygenated blood he needs while in the uterus, and (2) his mother may have a difficult time coping with the stress of labor. In essence, the baby will share his mother's problems; if she has congestive heart failure, so will he. Of course, the chances for a successful pregnancy depend on the severity of the condition, and as delivery draws near, the doctor may recommend a cesarian delivery or use forceps to make the birth less hazardous for mother and child.

Hypertension. When they become pregnant, women with high blood pressure may face problems similar to those of women with heart disease. It may be difficult for their bodies to supply all the oxygenated blood the fetus needs. Fetal oxygen deprivation during pregnancy may raise the chances of miscarriage, stillbirth, or neonatal death, but it is still true that the majority of women with treated, controlled hypertension do deliver normal babies. However, if a pregnant woman's blood pressure begins to rise, or her hypertension worsens, her doctor will almost certainly consider hospitalization so that she can be monitored and treated for preeclampsia, which sometimes follows high blood pressure.

Kidney disease. Kidney disease and its accompanying hypertension often preclude successful pregnancy, but some women with kidney disease—including some on kidney dialysis—have been able to carry a baby safely to term. Women with kidney disease may be advised to deliver by cesarean so as to spare both the mother and the child the stress of a prolonged labor.

Neurological Problems and Hormonal Imbalance

Both neurological impairment and hormonal imbalance may interfere with our reproductive functions.

To produce and maintain an erection, a man's body must be able to complete an intricate series of nerve impulses. Men with multiple sclerosis, spinal cord injuries or stroke-related disability may be unable to do this, or, if they attain erection, they may be unable to ejaculate. It's important to know, however, that the circumstances and results can differ dramatically from one person to another.

A woman whose lower body has been paralyzed either by a spinal cord injury or an illness such as polio may, if she becomes pregnant and carries her baby to term, be unable to muster the muscle action she needs to complete labor on her own. In such cases, an obstetrician is likely to advise a cesarian delivery.

Hormones are involved at every step in the reproductive process; any disorder of the pituitary, thyroid or hypothalamus (all of which release hormones that regulate our reproductive functions) can interfere with our ability to produce sperm or release a mature egg each month.

Phenylketonuria (PKU). People with PKU cannot metabolize the amino acid phenylalanine. As a result, it builds up in their bodies and, in newborns or young children, may damage brain cells. PKU, however, can be detected by simple blood or urine tests given right after the baby is born, thus allowing the doctor to put the infant on a special, protective diet.

According to recent research at the PKU clinic at Children's Hospital Medical Center in Boston, women who were PKU babies might do well to return to the special diet as soon as they become

pregnant so as to avoid the possibility of high levels of phenylalanine in their bodies damaging the fetus. In addition, in 1984, researchers at both MIT and the National Institute of Mental Health
suggested that it might be prudent for women who have PKU to
avoid the artificial sweetener aspartame while pregnant because the
aspartame degrades (breaks down) into several chemicals, including
phenylalanine. (See *30, Tests for the Newborn.*)

Rh incompatibility. When a woman with Rh-negative blood is
impregnated by a man whose blood is Rh-positive and the child they
conceive is Rh-positive, the woman's body will eventually produce
antibodies to destroy her baby's ''foreign'' red blood cells, much as
transplant patients produce antibodies to destroy transplanted tissues. Ordinarily, the production of antibodies doesn't take place
until after delivery, so the first child of an Rh-incompatible mother
and father is not likely to be affected. In order to protect future
children, an Rh-negative woman will be given an injection of Rh
antibodies within 72 hours after giving birth. These outside antibodies will keep the mother's body from producing its own antibodies. In effect, she will never be sensitized, which means that if
she conceives a second Rh-positive baby, she will not produce antibodies to destroy its red blood cells while she is pregnant. (Her
body will eliminate the outside antibodies within three to six months
after the injection, which should be repeated after every pregnancy
to protect the next child.)

Seizure disorders. Pregnant women with seizure disorders such
as epilepsy seem more likely to have babies with cardiac abnormalities. The drugs that control seizure disorders are also suspected
teratogens (substances that damage a developing fetus).

5. Do You Exercise?

As a general rule, women have more body fat than men do. The extra fat, concentrated at breast and hip, plays an important role in helping to maintain a woman's reproductive functions through her child-bearing years. After menopause, when the ovaries cease to produce a significant amount of estrogen, the extra body fat may serve as a source of the hormone.

When an otherwise healthy woman whose weight is within normal limits begins to lose large amounts of body fat through strict dieting or a strenuous exercise program, her menstrual periods may become irregular or she may cease to ovulate, which means that conception would be either difficult or impossible.

Clearly, this should not be interpreted to mean that all exercise is bad or that flab is fit. But the incidence of menstrual irregularities among ballet dancers or female runners is high enough to make it imperative that you never embark on a really heavy exercise regime without checking with your own doctor first. (To date, there are no studies showing any ill effects of strenuous exercise on the male reproductive system.)

As pregnancy begins to change the shape of your body you may decide to step up your regular exercise program. Labor will be hard work, and it certainly seems sensible to prepare for it by maintaining your muscle tone. But, while the mild stretching exercises included in most childbirth programs are useful, starting a new, strenuous exercise program when you become pregnant may be risky for your baby.

Exercise and the Fetal Oxygen Supply

When you work out, blood flows in greater quantities to the muscles you are using. Theoretically, this means that blood may be directed away from the vessels that supply the uterus, cutting down the flow of oxygen to the fetus. Because a number of studies of laboratory animals have shown that oxygen deprivation during pregnancy results in low-birthweight, deformed or stillborn infants, and some studies of human beings have suggested that the incidence of congenital heart defects rises along with the altitude at which a pregnant woman lives (there is less oxygen at high altitudes) and that pregnant marathoners are more likely than women who ease off on training while pregnant to produce small babies, the question of exercise during pregnancy is of some concern.

Exercise and Body Temperature

As a general rule, a normal, healthy human being has an internal body temperature of about 98.6°F (37°C). When you have a fever, your internal temperature goes up. It also goes up when you exercise or when you sit in a hot tub, sauna or steam room. (At the University of Washington Medical School, researchers found that sitting for 15 minutes in a tub filled with water heated to 102°F or for 10 minutes in a tub filled with water heated to 106°F could raise your body temperature to 102°F.) Throughout pregnancy, hyperthermia (a higher-than-normal body temperature) may be hazardous for the fetus. In one study of 113 aborted or miscarried embryos at Kyoto University in Japan, 18 percent of the women whose embryos had neural tube defects had had a fever early in pregnancy; only 4.9 percent of the women whose fetuses did not have neural tube defects had had a fever.

6. Are You under Emotional Stress?

Like physical stress, emotional stress has powerful effects on our bodies, including our reproductive systems. Under stress, some women find that their menstrual cycles become irregular or that they stop ovulating entirely for a while, and some studies suggest the possibility that women who are infertile or who have a history of miscarriage may be more anxious or emotionally troubled than other women. (Clearly, more research is needed to see which came first, the tendency to spontaneous abortion or the emotional stress.)

Men who are under stress may find it difficult (some would say impossible) to attain or maintain an erection, and there is some evidence to suggest that stress may also have some slight effects on sperm production. There's also some research suggesting that stress can change the environment of the vagina so that it isn't hospitable for sperm. Remember, though, that while stress may make it more difficult for you to conceive, pregnancy has occurred even in the most stressful conditions. Emotional stress is definitely *not* a means of birth control, but it may affect the course of a pregnancy.

When pregnant laboratory animals are exposed to the stress created by loud noise or high-frequency sound like the sound of a jet engine, they may produce low-birthweight offspring more frequently and there may be an increase in the numbers of infants born dead. In addition, when the high-frequency-sound exposure comes early in the animal's pregnancy, there may be an increased incidence of fetal death *in utero*.

In human beings, emotional stress may also play a role in damaging the fetus. At the Kaiser Foundation Health Plan in Oakland, California, researchers recently compiled information on fetal damage in 4,000 pregnancies occurring between 1959 and 1964, when abortion was not easily available. They found that women who did not want to be pregnant had a higher risk of spontaneous abortion than women who were pleased with their pregnancies. Infants born to women who had not wanted to be pregnant were one and a half times more likely to have a congenital abnormality, and researchers tentatively suggest that changes in hormonal levels caused by stress may have something to do with this.

7. Do You Smoke?

The Link to Conception

A 1981 study at Western General Hospital in Edinburgh, Scotland, suggests that men who smoke cigarettes are more likely than nonsmokers to produce abnormally shaped sperm. The researchers matched 43 smokers with 43 nonsmokers and found that the sperm samples from the smokers contained a significantly higher proportion of abnormal sperm—too large, too small, round-headed rather than oval, multiheaded or multitailed or immature. (There is some evidence that a sperm's shape reflects its genetic content. For example, men with cystic fibrosis, a genetic disorder, produce abnormally shaped sperm.) The Scottish study did not indicate how many years of smoking it takes to produce changes in sperm shapes or whether the men who smoked would produce normally shaped sperm if they stopped smoking.

Smoking and Fetal Damage

Unlike the evidence linking other addictive drugs to fetal damage, some of which is drawn from studies involving less than 30 infants, the evidence indicting nicotine is clear and unambiguous, drawn from more than 50 studies involving as many as half a million births.

Smoking affects the circulation of oxygen from mother to fetus. Nicotine is a vasoconstrictor. Every time you take a puff on your cigarette, your blood vessels—including the ones that supply the uterus—constrict for a moment, interrupting the flow of oxygenated blood to the baby. The burning cigarette also fills your blood with carbon monoxide that circulates to your baby and may depress its breathing each time you inhale. And, smoking may also damage your fetus's arteries. In 1981, using an electron microscope to examine the insides of umbilical arteries, a Dutch researcher found abnormal cells in the walls of umbilical arteries from women who smoked more than 10 cigarettes a day while pregnant. Presenting his findings to the Eighth European Cardiology Conference in Paris, he theorized that nicotine might make fetal arteries more porous, thus laying the foundation for arteriosclerosis (the abnormal buildup of fatty deposits in the arteries) later in life.

Babies born to women who smoke more than a pack of cigarettes a day while they are pregnant often are reported to weigh an average of 100–300 grams (3.3–10 oz.) less than babies born to women who do not smoke at all. Babies born to women who smoke less than a pack a day may also weigh less than babies born to women who don't smoke, but the difference between their weight and the "normal" birthweight is likely to be smaller.

Note that it isn't just a *mother's* cigarette smoke that may be hazardous for the fetus. In 1983, researchers at Cleveland Metropolitan General Hospital/Case Western Reserve University measured the levels of the tobacco-smoke by-product thiocyanate in the blood of more than 100 babies. Infants born to women who smoked during pregnancy had the highest levels of thiocyanate in their blood, but higher-than-normal levels of the chemical were also found in the blood of babies whose mothers were nonsmokers living with smokers.

The Evidence Against Smoking for Nursing Mothers

There is plenty of evidence to show that nursing mothers should not smoke. Nicotine may slow down the production of breast milk, reducing the supply available for your baby. The drug is excreted in breast milk, sometimes in concentrations high enough to irritate a nursing infant. And, if you or anyone else smokes while your baby is nursing or being fed, the infant may develop an aversion for whatever she is eating. During an experiment designed to explain food preferences in children, a psychologist at the New Mexico Institute of Mining and Technology found that laboratory mice exposed to cigarette smoke while drinking sweetened water avoided the sweetened water the next time it was offered. Perhaps babies who breathe in cigarette smoke while eating, particularly when they are tasting new foods, may decide that the food is unpleasant and turn it down the next time it is put on the table.

Part II

Sex

8. What Kind of Contraception Have You Used?

Like most other medical drugs or therapies, contraceptives can have unwelcome side effects. Some may make us less fertile even long after we stop using them. Others may harm a developing fetus if we inadvertently use them early in pregnancy or become pregnant while we are using them. Still others may harm a nursing infant if we use them while breast-feeding.

Contraceptives That May Make Us Less Fertile Even After We Stop Using Them

Women who use oral contraceptives are sometimes unable to conceive for a year or more after they give up The Pill. When ovulation and menstruation do start up again, the cycles may be irregular, and there have even been some reports of women who do not begin to ovulate or menstruate for as long as five years afterward.

IUDS may also affect fertility. These devices have been linked to a much-higher-than-normal incidence of pelvic inflammatory disease (PID), the infection that can scar the fallopian tubes and make it impossible for an egg to get through to meet the sperm. In one study, reported in *Family Planning Perspectives* in 1981, women who used IUDs were two times more likely than other women to be hospitalized for PID.

Other studies have shown similar results. In 1983, for example, researchers at Boston University School of Medicine reported in the *Journal of the American Medical Association* that women who use IUDs are nine times more likely than other women to develop a pelvic inflammation. The Boston researchers found that the risk appeared to vary according to which IUD the women chose.

Women who used the Dalkon shield seemed to have a risk 79 times higher than non-IUD users; women who used the Saf-T-Coil had a risk 24 times higher than non-IUD users; women who used the Lippes loop had a risk 13 times higher than women who used forms of contraception other than IUDs; and women who used a copper-impregnated IUD had a risk 7 times higher than women who did not use any IUD.

Contraceptives and Birth Defects

In April 1981, the *Journal of the American Medical Association* carried a study that seemed to suggest a link between vaginal spermicides and birth defects. The study was based on an analysis of the computer records of women who had belonged to a health cooperative in Seattle and were able to get contraceptive foams, jellies and creams free of charge. While the analysis did show a higher incidence of birth defects (shortened arms and legs, tumors, and chromosomal abnormalities, including Down's syndrome) among babies born to women who had gotten the spermicides through the cooperative, there was a problem with the data; the researchers had never talked to the women whose records they scrutinized. While they knew who had *gotten* the contraceptives, they didn't know for certain who had actually *used* them.

Since then, there have been several attempts to find out whether or not using vaginal spermicides raises the chances of having a child with birth defects. In 1982, for example, when researchers took a second look at the information they had gathered on more than 50,000 pregnancies for an earlier study on cerebral palsy, it turned out that 5 percent of the women who had told researchers that they used vaginal spermicides just before or just after they got pregnant did have babies with birth defects—but so did 4.5 percent of the women who didn't use foams, jellies and creams. Another 1982 report on more than 5,000 women who had used vaginal contraceptives just before or just after their last menstrual period (before they knew they were pregnant) showed the same thing. As yet, none of these studies is regarded as conclusive.

Does taking The Pill increase the chances of having a baby with birth defects? The evidence is contradictory. One study, in 1967, showed an increase in chromosomal abnormalities in the cells of women who had previously taken oral contraceptives, but there has not yet been any evidence of an increase in chromosomal abnormalities among babies born to these women than can be attributed directly to oral contraceptives. However, because of the possibility that The Pill may damage a fertilized egg, doctors advise that you stop taking oral contraceptives at least three months before becoming pregnant.

If a woman happens to take oral contraceptives very early in pregnancy, before she even knows that she has conceived, will the hormones in The Pill harm her baby? The evidence is mixed. Some studies appear to show a higher-than-normal incidence of malformations of the heart, limbs and neural tube in babies born to women who took oral contraceptives early in pregnancy, but other studies have failed to confirm this. Nonetheless, because it is well known that taking the sex hormones estrogen, diethylstilbestrol, progesterone or testosterone while you are pregnant can affect your baby's sex organs (masculinizing a female fetus or feminizing a male), the American Medical Association recommends that women stop taking The Pill as soon as pregnancy is confirmed.

Women who use the rhythm method or natural family planning have to be exceedingly careful in deciding when it is safe to have sex after the fertile period in the middle of the menstrual cycle. When a woman ovulates, the egg her ovary releases begins to move through the fallopian tubes and down into her uterus. If it isn't fertilized, it will eventually be expelled from her body. If she has sex several days after ovulation, but before the egg is gone, there is a chance that sperm may fertilize an "aging" egg ("delayed fertilization"). If that happens, there is an increased risk that the baby who is conceived will have chromosomal abnormalities or be spontaneously aborted. (See 9. *When and How Do You Make Love?*)

Contraceptives and Ectopic Pregnancy

If a fertilized egg implants and begins to grow anywhere outside the uterus, the resulting pregnancy is called ectopic (from the Greek word *ektopos*, "out of place"). On rare occasions, an ectopic pregnancy will go safely to term; healthy babies have been delivered alive after growing, for nine months, in their mothers' abdominal cavities. As a rule, however, ectopic pregnancies are generally considered highly dangerous because the most common place for them to occur is inside the fallopian tube, which would be ruptured as the baby grows.

If a woman becomes pregnant while using an IUD, her chances of having an ectopic pregnancy are eight times higher than they would be if she became pregnant while using another kind of contraceptive or no contraceptive at all. There are two reasons why this may be so. For one thing, the IUD protects approximately 98 percent against implantation of the fertilized egg in the uterus, but only 90 percent against implantation in another site, specifically, in the fallopian tube. Thus if pregnancy does occur, it's more likely to be somewhere other than the uterus (i.e., an ectopic pregnancy). Second, the progesterone in some IUDs may slow the fertilized and dividing egg's passage through the fallopian tubes so that it ends up implanting elsewhere.

How Contraceptives May Raise (or Lower) the Risk of an Infection While You Are Pregnant

An IUD is supposed to keep you from getting pregnant by keeping a fertilized egg from implanting in your uterus. However, if the IUD doesn't do its job and implantation occurs with the device in place (as it does to about 2 percent of all IUD users each year), there's about a 50 percent chance of a miscarriage. The highest risk of miscarriage among IUD users is linked to the higher rate of infection associated with IUDs.

If you plan to have intercourse while you are pregnant, your partner's using a condom may help lower your chances of developing an intercourse-related infection of the uterus. (See. 9. *When and How Do You Make Love?*)

Contraceptives and Breast-feeding

Folk medicine and an occasional scientific study sometimes suggest that nursing your baby is a natural form of contraception, but there is no conclusive evidence that lactation (producing milk) is a reliable way to keep from becoming pregnant.

If you start using oral contraceptives very soon after delivery, the hormones in The Pill may interfere with your production of milk and may affect the quality of the milk you do produce. The estrogen and progestins in oral contraceptives show up in breast milk. To date, there haven't been any problems reported in babies whose mothers were using The Pill while nursing, but the long-term effects are unknown.

9. When and How
Do You Make Love?

When you are trying to become pregnant, both the sexual position you choose and how frequently you have intercourse may affect your chances of conceiving.

After you become pregnant, whether or not you should continue to have intercourse is a question with both medical and psychological implications.

The Position That Makes Conception More Likely

The easier it is for the sperm to reach the egg, the more likely it is that you will get pregnant. You may increase your chances of conceiving, therefore, by using the classic "missionary" position, face-to-face with your partner on top. The reason why this position may be successful is obvious: when you lie on your back, with your knees drawn up and apart, your vaginal canal is shortened and sperm are deposited very close to the cervix.

How Often Should You Have Sex
When You Want To Have a Baby?

A normal, healthy man releases seminal fluid each time he has an orgasm, but the number of sperm in the fluid may fluctuate. The more frequently a man has an orgasm within a short period of time, the fewer sperm there will be in his ejaculate (seminal fluid). If your partner ordinarily has a low sperm count, or if you have been having difficulty conceiving, this may be crucial. It seems logical to have intercourse frequently when you are trying to become pregnant, but actually it may decrease your chances of conceiving. Some specialists, therefore, recommend having intercourse only once a day or once every 48 hours in the days right before ovulation.

The Safest Time to Have Sex When You Want to Conceive

As a mature egg makes its way from the ovary to the uterus, it "ages" (begins to deteriorate). For nearly 50 years scientists have known that fertilization of an aging egg results in a higher incidence of chromosomal abnormalities and Down's syndrome. It may also be linked to an increased incidence of spontaneous abortion. A 1975 study of 965 women who kept careful records of their monthly sexual activity showed that the probability of miscarriage went down significantly when pregnancy resulted from intercourse at the time of ovulation.* The chance of miscarriage tripled, however, when pregnancy resulted from intercourse three days *after* ovulation.

Is Sexual Intercourse During Pregnancy Linked to Uterine Infections?

Infections of the amniotic fluid inside the uterus are a leading cause of premature birth, as well as fetal or neonatal death. In one 1979 study of newborns, for example, 35 percent of the premature babies and 25 percent of the full-term infants who had respiratory problems also had infections of the amniotic fluid.

Many researchers, including Dr. Richard L. Naeye of Penn State's Milton S. Hershey Medical Center, suggest strongly that intercourse during pregnancy may be an important cause of these infections. They reason that seminal fluid released at ejaculation may loosen the layers of mucus that protect the cervix (the entrance to the uterus), thus allowing bacteria to enter the womb. Or, bacteria introduced into the vagina by the penis may proliferate in small

* The women recorded their basal temperature each day during the month and were able to pinpoint ovulation from this.

cracks in the surface of the lining of the vagina, and an infection may spread out from there.

According to Dr. Naeye, using condoms or washing the genitals thoroughly before having sex may help cut down the risk of an intercourse-related infection while you are pregnant (or even when you are not), but there is no way to eliminate it entirely.

Sexual Intercourse and Premature Labor

Many possibilities—including the physical pressure of the penis against the uterus and the contractions of orgasm—have been advanced to explain the apparent link between sexual intercourse during pregnancy and an increased incidence of premature delivery. One explanation popular right now has to do with prostaglandins, the natural chemicals we all manufacture inside our bodies. Some prostaglandins can cause the uterus to contract and may be used medically to induce abortion early in pregnancy. There are prostaglandins in male seminal fluid that some researchers believe may trigger premature labor following intercourse later in pregnancy.

Deciding Whether or Not to Have Sex While You Are Pregnant

Many women have continued to have intercourse during pregnancy without any ill effects for them or for their babies. So the real question is not whether or not having intercourse during pregnancy can cause problems—certainly in some cases it can—but whether or not it will cause problems for *you*.

Not surprisingly, there are several medical and physiological developments that may warn of trouble ahead. Ordinarily, your doctor may suggest that you might be safer refraining from intercourse during pregnancy

- if your cervix dilates easily or early
- if you have a history of miscarriage
- if the placenta is lying across the opening to the cervix (*placenta praevia*)
- If you or your partner have a chronic infection of the genitals

As research proceeds, and doctors learn more about the relationship between sexual intercourse during pregnancy and the safe delivery of a healthy baby, you can expect other risk factors to be identified.

Part III

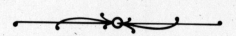

Drugs

10. Do You Use Illicit Drugs?

Many men who smoke marijuana claim that it increases sexual desire and improves sexual performance, but scientists who work with the drug have always had a hard time reconciling these anecdotal claims with studies that show how heavy use of marijuana may lower sperm counts and cause temporary impotence or infertility.

In 1983, researchers at the University of Texas Health Sciences Center in San Antonio came up with a possible solution to the puzzle. When they gave tetrahydrocannabinol (THC), the active ingredient in marijuana and hashish, to laboratory mice, they found that both high doses and low doses of THC caused a sudden rise in blood levels of two hormones, testosterone (the male sex hormone) and luteinizing hormone (LH), the hormone that triggers the release of a mature egg from the ovary in women and is linked to sperm production in men. As levels of the two hormones rose, the mice became more active sexually. After a while, though, in animals who had been given high doses of THC, the sudden rise in hormones was followed by an equally sudden decline. That seems to have some relationship to what has been observed in people: lowered sperm counts and other reproductive problems have turned up in men who use large amounts of marijuana (anywhere from 10 cigarettes a week to 20 a day), but no one has found these problems in men who use marijuana only sparingly.

In female laboratory animals, continued high doses of THC slow down ovarian function and lower the animals' body levels of LH and of follicle stimulating hormone (FSH). As yet, there is no proof that heavy use of marijuana produces the same effects in women, but it is known to disrupt menstrual cycles in women and in female laboratory animals. At the University of Maryland in 1983, for example, female monkeys given the equivalent of 15–18 marijuana cigarettes a week had irregular cycles for the first four months of the experiment. After that, the monkeys appeared to develop a tolerance for THC, and their cycles returned to normal.

The specific dose that produces menstrual irregularities in women isn't known.

Drugs and the Pregnant Woman

THC crosses the placenta from mother to fetus. When fed to pregnant laboratory animals or injected into them, THC has been linked to a slew of fetal defects, including retarded growth and malformation of the brain, spinal cord and limbs. In 1982, a team of researchers at Boston City Hospital found evidence to suggest that marijuana, as well as the marijuana user's life-style, may be hazardous to the fetus. Interviewing more than 1,600 women who had given birth at the hospital, the researchers discovered that babies born to women who had smoked marijuana three or more times a week while pregnant weighed an average of 4.6 ounces less at birth than babies born to women who did not use marijuana. And, marijuana seemed to multiply the effects of small amounts of alcoholic beverages. Women who drank very little while pregnant but also used marijuana had a fivefold increase in the incidence of babies born with fetal alcohol syndrome, the group of birth defects usually associated only with heavy drinking (i.e., more than 45 drinks a month (see 16. *What Do You Eat and Drink?*). However, the researchers pointed to the difficulty of isolating the effects of marijuana in these women, who also used other drugs and generally had poor nutritional habits (some said they ate only one or two meals a day while pregnant).

In 1972, the *Journal of the American Medical Association* carried the results of a study at George Washington University in Washington, D.C., attempting to assess the effects of LSD use on babies born to couples who had used the drug both *before* the baby was conceived and during pregnancy. Eight of 83 babies born alive to these couples had serious birth defects. While some women using LSD during pregnancy gave birth to healthy infants, three of the women who gave birth to defective infants had also used the drug while they were pregnant. In one case, only the father had used the drug, three days before the baby was conceived. In all the other cases, both mother and father had used LSD anywhere from three days to two years before conception. However, the researchers were unable to pin the birth defects specifically on LSD use because the people in the study had used a variety of other drugs, including marijuana, amphetamines, peyote and barbiturates, as well, and it was impossible to find a control group—people who had used all the other drugs but *no* LSD—with whom to compare the LSD users.

When given amphetamines, pregnant laboratory mice produced litters with defective hearts, eye problems and cleft palates. Women who used amphetamines while pregnant have delivered infants with deformed blood vessels.

Barbiturates cross the placenta. If you take a normal, therapeutic dose while you are pregnant, the concentration of the drug in your fetus's bloodstream will be equal to yours within three to five minutes. If you take an overdose, it may kill the fetus, which is unable to eliminate the drug efficiently. Barbiturates have been linked to birth defects in babies born to epileptic women, and babies born to women addicted to barbiturates are likely to be dependent on the drug themselves.

Heroin, methadone and morphine are opiods, a class of drugs that reduce pain, aggressive impulses and the desire for sex. If you use heroin while you are pregnant, it may slow down your baby's growth inside your womb. Morphine, which depresses breathing, can kill the fetus, and very large doses have been linked to abnormalities of the skeletal and cranial bones in the fetuses of pregnant animals. A pregnant woman who is addicted to heroin or methadone may go into premature labor if she tries to withdraw from the drug late in pregnancy (during the third trimester). Babies whose mothers are addicted to heroin, morphine or methadone may be born dependent on the drug and may show signs of withdrawal within one to seven days after they are born.

Drugs and the Nursing Mother

Clearly, nursing mothers should not be using illicit drugs. THC is excreted in breast milk. THC also lowers body levels of prolactin, the hormone that triggers milk production; whether smoking marijuana will actually make nursing more difficult remains to be proven.

Amphetamines, heroin, morphine, cocaine and barbiturates are also excreted in breast milk. If you use them while you are nursing, your baby will be getting them, too, and may suffer reactions similar to yours. For example, amphetamines in your milk can make your infant jittery; barbiturates can sedate her.

Illicit Drugs: Potential Problems for the Fetus

Drug	Hazardous for Animal Fetus	Hazardous for Human Fetus*	Babies Born to Women Who Use This Drug While Pregnant Are Likely to Be Addicted to or Dependent on the Drug
Amphetamines	Yes	Yes	No
Barbiturates	Yes	?†	Yes
Cocaine	No	?	No
Heroin	No	Yes	Yes
LSD	No	?	No
Marijuana	Yes	Yes	No
Methadone	Yes	?	Yes
Mescaline	Yes	?	No
Morphine	Yes	?	Yes

Sources: Gilman, Alfred Goodman; Goodman, Louis S.; Gilman, Alfred, eds., *The Pharmacological Basis of Therapeutics,* 6th ed. (Macmillan, 1980); Martin, Eric, *The Hazards of Medication* (Lippincott, 1978); Shepard, Thomas H., *Catalogue of Teratogenic Agents,* 4th ed. (Johns Hopkins, 1983).

* Refers to birth defects, toxicity, growth retardation and other damage; excludes potential addiction.

† means either that studies have shown conflicting evidence or that no studies have been done.

11. Are You Taking Medication?

Many well-known, frequently prescribed drugs interfere with our sexuality or our reproductive functions. Some of these drugs increase or decrease our interest in sex. Others make it difficult, if not impossible, for a man to have an erection, or they may impede ejaculation or delay orgasm. Some drugs slow down the production of sperm or make sperm less active, thus reducing their chances of reaching and penetrating a mature egg. And some drugs disrupt a woman's menstrual cycle, making it hard for her to predict with any certainty when she will be ovulating and able to conceive.

Some of these sexual and reproductive side effects are painfully obvious to the people involved; others have been observed only in research on laboratory animals. Most studies on the sexual dysfunction and reproductive problems that may result from drug therapy only mention the things that happen to men. Sexual side effects in women, such as painful intercourse caused by a vaginal infection after antibiotic therapy, rarely receive the same attention. If you have any symptoms like this after using a prescription or nonprescription drug, let your doctor know right away.

Many otherwise useful and effective drugs cross the placenta and may endanger a developing fetus. That is why no pregnant woman should ever take a drug that has not been specifically prescribed by her doctor. On the other hand, it is important to remember that some drugs are vital, even though they may have side effects. Please consider this warning very carefully:

Never, under any circumstances, stop taking a drug your doctor has prescribed for you while you are pregnant without discussing it with him first. It is true that some of the drugs you are taking may be dangerous for the fetus, but it is also true that some of the conditions for which they are prescribed may also be hazardous to your baby. This warning assumes that your doctor knew that you were pregnant when he pre-

scribed the drug or knows that you have since conceived. Obviously, it is essential that you tell him as quickly as possible when you know—or suspect—that you have conceived because this may affect his decision in prescribing a drug or course of treatment for you. This warning applies not just to your obstetrician but to any doctor who prescribes medicine for you.

As you approach delivery, prescription and nonprescription drugs continue to be of concern. Childbirth is a natural function, and if everything goes smoothly you may be able to deliver your baby without the help of anesthetics or other drugs. But it's important to remember that "natural" doesn't always mean "perfect." Emergencies happen when babies are being born, and there are times when the right drug can make a difficult or dangerous labor safer and less stressful.

The key to a successful delivery may well be the decision you make months or even years before you get to the delivery room, when you choose your obstetrician. Having chosen someone whose medical opinions you know and share will give you the freedom to trust him or her to use judiciously every tool available, including obstetrical drugs. It's true that many, if not all, of these drugs may have side effects for you and for your baby, but just as you would not avoid using the medication you need while you are pregnant, you should not refuse out of hand to consider these drugs that may relax the uterus, help labor along or make the delivery more comfortable for you and for your baby.

Finally, when talking about drugs, remember that it's a virtual certainty that any drug you take while you are nursing will eventually show up in your milk.

Drugs That Affect Libido

Libido is the desire for sex. Some drugs, such as sedatives and tranquilizers, reduce libido simply by making us sleepy or depressed. Others, such as the ulcer drug *cimetadine* (TAGAMET), which inactivates male hormones, or *propranalol* (INDERAL), which blocks the reception of some chemical signals inside the body, can break the chain of chemical commands that trigger desire. Cancer drugs that damage ovaries or testes may also reduce libido.

Drugs That May Affect Libido

Antidepressants

Amitriptyline (ELAVIL), amoxapine (ASENDIN), desipramine (BORPRAMIN, PERTOFRANE), doxepin (SINEQUAN), imipramine (TOFRANIL)

Antihypertensives

Methyldopa (ALDOMET), prazosin (MINIPRESS), propranolol (INDERAL), reserpine (SANDRIL, SERPASIL), spironolactone (ALDACTONE)

Glaucoma medication

Acetazolamide (AKZOL, DIAMOX), dichlorphenamide (DARANIDE), methazolamide (NEPTAZINE)

Tranquilizers

Alprazolam (XANAX), chlordiazepoxide (LIBRAX, LIBRIUM, LIBRITABS, LIMBRITOL), diazepam (VALIUM), haloperidol (HALDOL), oxazepam (SERAX), reserpine, triflupromazine (VESPRIN)

Sources: AMA Drug Evaluations, 5th ed., (American Medical Association, 1983); Lee, I.P., *Effects of Drugs and Chemicals on Male Reproduction* (National Institute of Environmental Health Sciences, 1981); *The Medical Letter,* August 5, 1983; *The Physicians' Desk Reference,* 36th ed. (Medical Economics Company, 1982).

Drugs That May Cause Impotence, Interfere with Ejaculation, or Delay Orgasm

Some drugs interrupt the complicated series of nerve and muscle impulses and reactions that make erection, ejaculation and orgasm possible. Antihypertensives and drugs such as sedatives, tranquilizers, or antidepressants that affect the central nervous system are all capable of interfering with erection or ejaculation. (While it is not absolutely necessary for a man to have an erection in order to deposit sperm into the vaginal tract, without ejaculation conception is impossible.)

Amphetamines and the antidepressant *imipramine* (IMIVATE, TOFRANIL) may delay orgasm in women; *desipramine* (NORPRAMIN), another antidepressant, has been reported to produce this effect in men.

Drugs That May Cause Impotence, Ejaculatory Problems or Delayed Orgasm

Antidepressants
Amitriptyline (ELAVIL, ENDEPT, ENOVIL), amoxipine (ASENDIN), desipramine (NORPRAMIN), doxipin (ADAPIN, SINEQUAN), imipramine (IMIVATE, TOFRANIL), nortriptyline (AVENTIL, PAMELOR), phenelzine (NARDIL), protriptyline (VIVACTIL), tranylcypromine (PARNATE), trazadone (DESYREL), trimipramine (SURMONTIL)

Antialcoholism medication
Disulfiram (ANTABUSE)

Antihypertensives
Clonidine (CATAPRES), guanethidine (ESIMIL), labetalol (TRANDATE, VESCOL), methyldopa (ALDOMET), prazosin (MINIPRESS), spironolactone (ALDACTONE), timolol (BLOCADREN)

Cough medicine
Potassium iodate

*Antispasmodics**
Anisotropine (VALPIN), clidinium (QUARZAN), isopromide iodide (DARBID), mepenzolate (CANTIL), methantheline (BANTHINE), oxyphenonium bromide (ANTRENYL), tridihexethyl chloride (PATHILON)

Glaucoma medication
Acetazolamide (AK-ZOL, DIAMOX), dichlorphenamide (DARANIDE, ORATROL), methazolamide (NAPTAZANE)

Tranquilizers
Haloperidol (HALDOL),† lithium (LITHANE, LITHOBID, LITHONATE, LITHOTABS, PFI-LITH), mesoridazine (SERENTIL), piperacetazine (MELLARIL)

Ulcer medication
Cimetidine (TAGAMET)

Sources: *AMA Drug Evaluations,* 5th ed. (American Medical Association, 1983); Lee, I.P., *Effects of Drugs and Chemicals on Male Reproduction* (National Institute of Environmental Health Sciences, 1981); *The Physicians' Desk Reference,* 36th ed. (Medical Economics Company, 1982).
* In large doses.
† Also used as an antiemetic, a drug to control vomiting.

Drugs That May Make a Man Infertile

In men, potency is the ability to have an erection and consummate sexual intercourse; fertility is the ability to provide sperm that can fertilize a waiting egg. For a man to be fertile, his semen must contain a normal amount of healthy, active sperm, but "normal" is a relative term. A man whose sperm count is slightly lower than it should be won't necessarily be infertile since nature provides a generous margin for error. So long as his sperm are healthy and able to move about, conception may be possible. (See *22. Tests That Measure Fertility.*)

Some drugs reduce fertility by slowing the production of sperm or halting it altogether; others may damage sperm so that they cannot move about actively. Still others may kill the sperm in the semen. A man who has less than a normal amount of sperm in his semen suffers from oliogospermia; a man with no living sperm in his semen suffers from azoospermia.

Some Drugs That Interfere with Sperm Production or Damage Sperm in the Semen

---

Anticancer drugs
Busulfan (MYLERAN), chlorambucil (LEUKERAN), cyclophosphamide (CYTOXAN, NEOSPAR), methotrexate, mechlorethamine (MUSTARGEN)

Anti-inflammatory agents
Sulfasalazine (AZULSAFADINE)

Gout medication
Colchicine (COLBENEMIDE, COL-PROBENECID)

Urinary tract antiseptics
Nitrofuradantoin (FURADANTIN, MACRODANTIN), trimethoprim-sulfamethoxazole (BACTRIM, SEPTRA)

Sources: *AMA Drug Evaluations,* 5th ed. (American Medical Association, 1983); "Drug information forum," *U.S. Pharmacist,* December 1982; Lee, I.P., *Effects of Drugs and Chemicals on Male Reproduction* (National Institute of Environmental Health Sciences, 1981); *The Physicians' Desk Reference,* 36th ed. (Medical Economics Company, 1982).

Drugs That Affect the Menstrual Cycle

Several anticancer drugs and a number of tranquilizers appear to cause irregular menstruation. Sometimes ovulation stops altogether until the drug is discontinued. Women whose cycles are very irregular will find it difficult to predict when ovulation is likely to occur; women who do not ovulate cannot become pregnant.

Some Drugs That May Disrupt the Menstrual Cycle

Anticancer drugs
Busulfan (MYLERAN), chlorambucil (LEUKERAN), cyclophosphamide (CYTOXAN, NEOSAR), thiotepa

Corticosteroids
ACTH (ACTHAR)

Tranquilizers
Alprazolam (XANAX), chlordiazepoxide (LIBRAX, LIBRIUM, LIBRITABS, LIMBRITOL), thioradazine (MELLARIL), triflupromazine (VESPRIN)

Sources: *AMA Drug Evaluations,* 5th ed. (American Medical Association, 1983); *The Physicians' Desk Reference,* 36th ed. (Medical Economics Company, 1982).

Drugs That May Damage Chromosomes

Can prescription or nonprescription drugs cause birth defects by damaging sperm or ova before conception occurs? An increasing number of medical drugs are now known to damage (break) chromosomes, and many experts suspect that these drugs may cause birth defects in infants that result from the fertilization of an egg by a drug-damaged spermatozoon. However intriguing this possibility may be, to date it has not been proven by scientifically designed studies.

Classifying Prescription and Nonprescription Drugs for Pregnant Women

Even though it is now clear how and when many prescription and nonprescription drugs may injure a developing fetus, it is still impossible to put together a complete list of all the medications that may be hazardous to your baby.

There are several reasons for this lingering uncertainty. First, many of our most popular medicines have been around for decades. They were introduced before the Food and Drug Administration set up its now-stringent regulations for testing drugs, and our information about them comes from experience, not controlled tests. Second, even the drugs that now go through multiple tests before they are put on the market may not show their true colors before they are released for sale. Animals and human beings do not always react the same way; one species in a test series may react the way people do while another species doesn't, which is why it is extremely important for researchers to test the drugs on as many species of animals as possible.

To deal with the uncertainty, the FDA has created five categories to describe a drug's relative safety during pregnancy. These descriptions are now included as part of the labeling information for every prescription drug. You will find them in the small booklet (the "package insert") that comes with your medicine:

Category A applies to drugs for which controlled studies in women fail to demonstrate a risk to the fetus. Even though it is impossible to say that these drugs will never be hazardous for the developing fetus, a "reasonable presumption" of safety is possible. Like all other drugs, they should be used during pregnancy only when they are really needed.

Category B means either that animal studies haven't shown any problems but that there aren't adequate studies on human beings, or that animal studies *have* shown a risk confirmed in controlled studies on women.

Category C means either that animal studies have shown a problem but there are no adequate, controlled studies on women, or that there are no studies available either for animals or human beings.

Category D applies to drugs that have been shown to be linked to birth defects in human beings but which provide potential benefits that make them useful despite their known risks. These are drugs that may be useful in life-threatening situations or to treat serious diseases for which no safe drug exists. If you have to use one of these drugs, your doctor should tell you about the risks it poses for your baby.

Category X drugs are the ones whose ability to damage or destroy the fetus have been clearly demonstrated in animal or human studies and whose risks outweigh their benefits. These drugs should not be used while you are pregnant.

Drugs Reported to Be Hazardous to the Fetus

Analgesics. Several common painkillers appear to be dangerous for the fetus if you take them while you are pregnant.

Aspirin is an anticoagulant. It crosses the placenta. Taken during the last week or so before delivery it may cause bleeding problems for both mother and child during labor. Because it is difficult, if not impossible, to pinpoint the delivery date in advance, most doctors simply recommend avoiding aspirin entirely during the third trimester of pregnancy. Others suggest avoiding it throughout pregnancy because, in addition to its being linked to bleeding problems at delivery, aspirin may also prolong labor, contribute to the birth of a low-birthweight infant or be implicated in the development of a severe form of neonatal jaundice that can damage a newborn baby's brain. (Note: Many otherwise healthy babies do develop an unrelated, mild jaundice that goes away quickly in the first few days of life.)

Acetaminophen and *propoxyphene* (DARVON and related products) also cross the placenta. Acetaminophen has been found in the urine of newborns whose mothers used the drug while pregnant, but there haven't been any well-controlled, formal studies of the effects of either drug during pregnancy.

Indomethacin (INDOCIN) and *naproxen* (NAPROSYN), nonsteroidal, anti-inflammatory analgesics, also cross the placenta. In animal tests, these two have been shown to cause the *ductus arteriosus* (an opening from the fetal heart into the fetus's major artery which normally stays open until the baby is born) to close prematurely, before birth. The result is a reduced circulation of fetal blood.

Acne medication. *Isotretinoin* (ACCUTANE) is a vitamin A derivative given orally for the treatment of severe acne. In 1983, it was reported to have been linked to deformities of the central nervous system in three babies whose mothers had used the drug while they were pregnant.

Antacids and ulcer drugs. The safety of antacids during pregnancy has not been established. In one study asking new mothers what drugs they had taken while they were pregnant, there seemed to be a higher incidence of babies with both major and minor malformations born to women who had used antacids early in pregnancy, but there has been no follow-up on this and no single antacid was implicated.

Antibiotics. Amikacin (AMIKIN), *gentamycin* (APOGEN, BRISTA-GEN, GARAMYCIN) *kanamycin* (KANTREX), *streptomycin* and *tobramycin* (NEBCIL) are aminoglycosides, a group of antibiotics that can damage hearing. During pregnancy, streptomycin can damage the fetus's auditory nerves, and it is suspected that the other aminoglycosides may, too. Taken early in pregnancy, streptomycin may cause multiple malformations, include micromelia (disproportionately small arms and legs).

Sulfa drugs may be hazardous late in pregnancy. If taken during the third trimester, they may contribute to the development of a severe form of neonatal jaundice that can damage a baby's brain. *Trimethoprim,* which is sometimes combined with the sulfa drug *sulfasoxazole* as a urinary tract antiseptic (BACTRIM, SEPTRA), has caused malformations in the fetuses of pregnant laboratory animals.

Tetracyclines all cross the placenta and end up in the fetus' bones and in the small buds that will eventually become her teeth.

Tetracyclines may retard the growth of fetal bones and can cause permanent brownish-yellow staining of the teeth.

Anticoagulants. *Dicumarol* and *warfarin* (ATHROMBIN, COUMADIN, PANWARFIN), coumarin derivatives, cross the placenta and have been linked to a number of fetal malformations and defects. Taken between the sixth and the ninth weeks of pregnancy, coumarin derivatives may cause fetal warfarin syndrome (facial malformations and deformities of the long bones that can cause reduced height or weight) or scoliosis (curvature of the spine). Taken during the second and third trimesters, coumarin derivatives have been linked to problems with the central nervous system: mental retardation, blindness, spasticity, seizures.

Anticonvulsants. Despite the fact that both anticonvulsants and the seizure disorders they are used to treat may increase the chances of delivering a baby with congenital malformations or mental defects, the fact is that women who must use these drugs while pregnant still have a 90 percent chance of producing a completely normal baby.

Trimethadione (TRIDONE), perhaps the most dangerous of the anticonvulsants, is a rarely used drug. According to data reported by the American Medical Association, up to 80 percent of the embryos exposed to this drug were either spontaneously aborted or born with birth defects.

Late in 1982, the Centers for Disease Control in Atlanta, Georgia, reported that information from a French center for the study of birth defects appeared to show a significantly higher risk for babies born to women who used the anticonvulsant *valproic acid* (DEPAKNE) during the first three months of pregnancy.

Phenobarbital and *phenytoin* (DILANTIN), two other anticonvulsants, may be linked to congenital malformations (abnormalities of the head, face and limbs), mental retardation, or coagulation problems in the newborn. And, phenytoin may slow down the fetus's normal growth in the womb.

Antidepressants. There have been reports of congenital malformations in a number of infants whose mothers took the tricyclic antidepressants *desipramine* (NORPRAMIN, PERTOFRANE) and *imip-*

ramine (TOFRANIL) while they were pregnant, but there haven't been any well-controlled studies to determine whether there was a cause-and-effect relationship between the drugs and the birth defects. Another tricyclic antidepressant, *amoxipine* (ASENDIN), caused low birthweight, fetal death and stillbirth among the fetusus of pregnant laboratory animals given doses 3 to 10 times the normal human dose. There is no information as to the ultimate safety of these or any of the other tricyclic antidepressants during pregnancy.

Another antidepressant, *trazodone* (DESYRYL) has caused an increased rate of fetal resorption (the fetus is reabsorbed into the mother's body) in laboratory rats and congenital birth defects in rabbits. There are no studies of its effects on human beings.

Antiprotozoals. *Metronidazole* (FLAGYL, METRYL), used to treat *Trichomonas* infections and amebiasis (an infection caused by the parasite *Entamoeba histolytica*), is a mutagen, a substance that can change the genetic material in living cells. It crosses the placenta, and, while no adverse effects on the fetus have been reported to date, this drug is usually avoided druing the first three months of pregnancy.

Quinine, used to treat malaria, can damage the fetus's auditory nerve and is suspected of causing miscarriage and general malformations. So is its pharmaceutical cousin, *chloroquine*.

Antispasmodics. *Atropine, belladonna* and *dicyclomine*—all of which may be used to treat irritable bowel syndrome—show mixed results. In each case, one study showed evidence of malformations, while another showed none. Since all the studies centered on very small groups of patients, no conclusions could be drawn, and the safety or lack of it for these drugs during pregnancy has not been established.

Antiworm drugs *(anthelmintics)*. Large doses of *metrofonate* (BILARCIL) caused changes in chromosomes in animal tests. *Niridazole* (AMBILHAR) is also mutagenic. *Hycanthone mesylate* (ETRENOL) is mutagenic and carcinogenic in animals and has also caused fetal malformations. *Mebendazole* (VERNOX) has caused malformations in the fetuses of pregnant laboratory rats, but not in dogs, sheep or horses. *Quinacrine* (ATRABRINE), which may (rarely) cause aplastic anemia and liver damage, is known to cross the placenta.

Asthma drugs. As of this writing, there haven't been any reports of malformations in babies born to women who used the bronchodilators (drugs that open up the air passages in our lungs) *aminophylline* and *theophylline* while they were pregnant. However, sometimes babies born to these women had temporary fast heartbeat or were jittery at birth.

The asthma preventive *cromolyn sodium* (INTAL) has been linked to a higher rate of fetal resorption and low birthweight among infants born to laboratory animals given doses high enough to be toxic to the mothers. There is no evidence of any such effect in such women given normal doses of this drug.

Cancer drugs. Of all the drugs in common use today, the ones most likely to cause malformations of the fetus are the antioplastics, drugs that keep cancer cells from developing, maturing or spreading. Yet the good news is that in 9 out of 10 pregnancies allowed to come to term after a pregnant woman has taken one of these drugs, a normal infant is born. If you become pregnant while you are under treatment for cancer, your doctor can give you more detailed information on any risks your baby may face.

Diuretics. Some diuretics may be hazardous to a developing fetus. For example, when pregnant rats were given doses of *acetazolamide* 10 times higher than those commonly used for people, they gave birth to infants without forelimbs (no such problem showed up in pregnant laboratory rabbits given the same drug).

The thiazide diuretics (*bendroflumethiazide, benzthiazide, chlorothiazide, cyclothiazide, hydrochlorothiazide,* and so on) may be linked to low birthweight, fetal hypoglycermia and neonatal jaundice.

Furosemide may alter the levels of sodium and uric acid in the fetus's blood, and all diuretics may affect the flow of liquids across the placenta.

For all these reasons, many doctors prefer not to use diuretics to treat the uncomplicated water retention that is so common in pregnancy. No such compunction exists when it comes to treating hypertension that does not respond to other means or medications. Because the effects of untreated hypertensions may be so devastating for both mother *and* child, the possible risk of treatment with the diuretics may be considered justified.

Douches. Some douches contain *povidone-iodine,* an antiseptic that may be absorbed through the mother's vaginal walls and passed through the placenta to the fetus. The iodine may suppress the fetus's production of thyroid hormones.

Hormones. If taken by a pregnant woman during the first three months of pregnancy, androgens (male hormones) and progestins (protesterone) can masculinize a female fetus's external genitals, enlarging the clitoris to the size of a small penis.

If taken by a pregnant woman at any time during her pregnancy, *diethystilbesterol* (DES), a synthetic estrogen, may cause vaginal tumors and malformations of the uterus and cervix in female children and malformations of the genitals in males. (These tumors and malformations may not be apparent for years after the baby is born.)

Women who take oral contraceptives very early in pregnancy, before they even know they are pregnant, may have an increased risk of delivering a baby with birth defects, but the evidence of this is contradictory. (See *8. What Kind of Contraception Do You Use?*)

Very large doses of corticosteroids (*cortisone, hydrocortisone*) taken by a pregnant woman may shrink the fetus's adrenal glands so that they cannot produce adequate supplies of these hormones for the baby. (See also *Thyroid medication,* p. 54.)

Hypertension medication. Like many other useful and effective drugs, *methyldopa* (ALDOMET) crosses the placenta. To date, no unusual or teratogenic effects on the fetus have been reported.

Metoprolol (LOPRESSOR) and *propranolol* (INDERAL) both cross the placenta. Propranolol has been associated with fetal growth retardation, depressed breathing in the newborn and an increased incidence of death soon after birth.

Reserpine is the only hypertensive drug that is suspected of causing malformations in the fetus. In the newborn it may cause nasal discharge, stuffiness and obstruction that is sometimes severe enough to be fatal. This drug is rarely used in pregnancy except to treat eclamptic women. (See also *Diuretics,* p. 52.)

Migraine remedies. Products containing ergot derivatives are never used for a pregnant woman because ergot causes uterine contractions and may trigger a miscarriage. The following drugs contain ergot derivatives: BELLERGAL, CAFERGOT, CAFERGOT P-B, D.H.E. 45, ERGOMAR, ERGOSTAT, GYNERGEN, MIGRAL, SANSERT, WIGRAINE. FIORINAL does not contain an ergot derivative, but it does contain a barbiturate, *butalbital.* (See *Sedatives,* below.)

Sedatives and tranquilizers. While barbiturates are suspected teratogens, studies of their effects during pregnancy are contradictory. They are known to cross the placenta and may depress the fetus's breathing and its central nervous system. Babies born to women who are dependent on barbiturates or use them heavily in the last trimester of pregnancy may themselves be dependent.

In 1974, a study of 19,044 newborns appeared to show that babies whose mothers had used either *meprobamate* (MILTOWN, EQUANIL) or chlordiazepoxide (LIBRIUM) during the first six weeks of pregnancy had a sharply increased risk of birth defects; 5 of the 66 babies born to women who had used meprobamate had congenital heart defects. However, a second study the following year was unable to confirm these results.

Chlordiazepoxide is one of the benzodiazepine tranquilizers, a groups of drugs that includes *diazepam* (VALIUM), *flurazepam* (DALMANE), oxazepam (SERAX), and prazepam (CENTRAX), among others. A woman dependent on one of these drugs or using it heavily during the last three months of pregnancy, may give birth to a drug-dependent child. In addition, chlordiazepoxide, diazepam and oxazepam were suspected of causing cleft lip and/or cleft palate if used early in pregnancy. This suspicion has not been confirmed and, indeed, has been disputed in several recent studies.

Thyroid medication. Radioactive iodides that are used to treat hyperthyroidism (an overactive thyroid gland) can cross the placenta and destroy the fetus's thyroid. Other drugs used to treat hyperthyroidism may interfere with the fetus's own normal production of thyroid hormones, but thyroid hormones used to treat an underactive thyroid (hypothyroidism) will not cross the placenta and cannot affect the baby.

Tuberculosis drugs. In 1979, an article in *Teratology,* a journal devoted to information about substances that can damage the developing fetus, reported five cases of brain damage in infants whose mothers had been given *isoniazid* (DOW-ISONIAZID, NYDRAZID) while pregnant. However, the article's author suggests that the damage may actually have been due to a vitamin B_6 deficiency, since our bodies excrete more vitamin B_6 than normal when we metabolize isoniazid.

There has been one report of a newborn and its mother having suffered liver and bleeding difficulties after the mother used *rifampin* (RIFADIN, RIMACTANE) while pregnant. (See also *Antibiotics,* p. 49.)

Drugs That Relax the Uterus and Help Postpone Labor

If you go into labor prematurely, your doctor may try to halt your contractions with a drug that relaxes the uterus. Among the drugs used to halt premature labor are *beta*-adrenergics, intravenous alcohol, magnesium sulfate and prostaglandin inhibitors.

There is no scientific study to show exactly how reliable these drugs are, but when they do work they can help to put off delivery for anywhere from a few hours to a few weeks, giving your baby some more time in which to mature in the womb. During this time, your doctor may give you steroid hormones such as *hydrocortisone* that help to accelerate the development of your baby's lungs (a premature baby's immature lungs often fail to function outside his mother's womb).

Not every woman will respond to these drugs, nor is every woman a good candidate for them. To benefit, a woman must be less than 34 weeks pregnant (doctors usually go ahead and deliver an infant who has spent at least 34 weeks in the womb), her membranes must be intact, and her cervix cannot be fully dilated. If she has bleeding or heart disease, or if there is an inflammation caused by an infection of the amniotic sac, her doctor will ordinarily not attempt to halt labor.

Beta-adrenergics relax smooth muscles by changing muscle cells so that they will not accept chemical signals telling them to contract. The *beta*-adrenergic currently used to relax the uterus and halt premature labor is *ritodrine* (YUTOPAR). Because there is no evidence to show whether or not it causes birth defects if given early in pregnancy, ritodrine is never used before the twentieth week. Its possible side effects include low blood pressure and a faster heartbeat for the mother, a faster heartbeat for the baby, and higher levels of insulin in the umbilical cord that may cause hypoglycemia in the newborn. To date follow-up studies on babies whose mothers were given ritodrine do not show any problems later in life.

Other *beta*-adrenergics that may halt premature contractions but have not yet been approved for this purpose are *albuteral* (PROVENTIL, VENTOLIN), *terbutaline sulfate* (BRICANYL, BRETHINE) and several other drugs currently being used as bronchodilators.

Alcohol given intravenously can keep the pituitary from releasing oxytocin, a hormone that causes the uterus to contract. (See *Drugs That Stimulate Uterine Contractions during Labor,* p. 57.) Intravenous alcohol may postpone labor for a few hours or days. It can cause inebriation in both mother and child, and some experts recommend against its use.

Magnesium sulfate, like the *beta*-adrenergics, keeps muscle cells from reacting to chemical signals ordering them to contract. This drug is used to prevent convulsions and uterine contractions in women with pre-eclampsia; it has not yet been approved for halting premature labor in women who are not pre-eclamptic. Its side effects include weakened tendon responses in the mother and weakened muscle responses in the baby. It is never used for women with heart disease or kidney problems.

Prostaglandin inhibitors keep the uterus from releasing prostaglandins that cause it to contract. Some prostaglandin inhibitors have been approved for use in treating menstrual cramps caused by an overproduction of prostaglandins, but they haven't yet been approved for halting premature labor.

Drugs That Stimulate Uterine Contractions During Labor

Drugs that make your uterus contract can be used to induce labor, strengthen your own natural contractions or tighten your uterus and reduce uterine bleeding after your baby is born. Oxytocin is commonly used for inducing labor and strengthening the contractions; ergot drugs are commonly used to tighten the uterus after birth.

Oxytocin is a hormone produced in your hypothalamus and stored in your pituitary. Since your pituitary continues to release oxytocin all during your pregnancy, exactly how it signals the start of labor is still a mystery, although some researchers suggest that the uterus simply becomes more sensitive to its effects later in pregnancy.

Synthetic oxytocin may be used to bring on labor when there is an important reason to help the baby out of the womb as quickly as possible. For example, the membranes may have ruptured prematurely, exposing the baby to infection. Or, there may be bleeding or complications of diabetes or pre-eclampsia. Or, the placenta may no longer be capable of providing the oxygen and nutrients the baby needs. Some doctors use oxytocin to induce labor when a pregnancy has gone on longer than 42 weeks; others prefer to wait for a child who is alive and healthy in the womb to move on her own.

During labor, if a woman's contractions have slackened or are simply not strong enough to help her child down the birth canal, her doctor may use oxytocin to make them more effective.

Doctors usually will not attempt to bring on labor or make the contractions stronger if

- the baby's head is very large
- the baby is lying in a position other than "head down"

- previous deliveries were by cesarean section
- the cervix is weakened by scarring
- the placenta, instead of sitting in its normal position at the top of the uterus, is lying across the bottom, blocking the exit through the cervix, a condition known as *placenta praevia.*

Ergot is produced by a fungus that grows on rye. For more than 2,000 years, people have known that it causes strong contractions of the uterus, but it was not until the 1800s that doctors began to use it as an obstetrical drug. (Folk medicine practitioners or herbalists had sometimes used it as an abortifacient, a role in which it is exceedingly dangerous and potentially lethal.)

Today, the ergot derivatives *ergotamine tartrate, ergonovine* (ERGOTRATE) and *methylergonovine* (METHERGINE) may be used to make the uterus contract after the placenta has been delivered, thus cutting down the chances of hemorrhage. The effects of these drugs may last for several hours, which is why they are never used to bring on labor or strengthen natural contractions. Their possible side effects include hypertension (with nausea, vomiting, blurred vision and headaches), convulsions and death.

NOTE: Prostaglandins also cause the uterus to contract. Right now, the prostaglandins *carboprost* (PROSTIN/15M), *dinoprost* (PROSTIN F2 ALPHA) and *dinoprostone* (PROSTIN E2) are used in second-trimester abortions and to stimulate uterine contractions in incomplete miscarriage or when the baby has died in the womb. It is possible that in the future these drugs will also be used either to stimulate contractions during labor or to help the uterus contract after delivery.

Drugs That Relieve Pain and Stress During Childbirth

None of the anesthetics used to make labor or delivery less painful are completely safe for the baby. According to the Food and Drug Administration, every one of them can decrease the baby's muscle tone or ability to suck, make him less responsive to all kinds of stimulation, slow down his breathing and make his heartbeat irregular. All these effects are short-term, likely to disappear within a few days after birth, but right now there is virtually no information about the possible long-term effects of anesthetics used during delivery.

As a result, many women refuse to consider any painkillers at all while they are in labor. But it is important to remember that stress, pain and anxiety may cause your body to produce chemicals that slow down the flow of blood to the uterus, which means that your baby may get less oxygen than he needs. Some of us can deal with the stress of labor through routines such as the Lamaze method that offer a kind of psychological anesthesia. These methods will not work for everyone, though, or they may not work through the

---

Procedures Using Local Anesthetics

Pudendal block	Anesthetic is injected directly into the tissues in the genital area. It will block the pain of low forceps or an episiotomy, but won't relieve the pain of contractions or make them weaker.
Paracervical block	Anesthetic is injected into tissue around the cervix. It will block sensation in this area, but it has to be repeated several times during labor. Up to 70% of the babies born to mothers who have had paracervical blocks have a slow heartbeat.
Caudal block	Anesthetic is injected into the spinal column below the spinal cord. The drug will cross through the *dura mater* (the hard membrane covering the cord) and anesthesize nerves in the lower part of the body so that you cannot "push." High concentrations show up in your bloodstream, cross to the baby, and may affect her for as long as 48 hours after birth.
Lumbar epidural block	"Epidural" means "outside the *dura*." This form of anesthesia is similar to a caudal block except that the anesthetic is injected higher in the spinal column and affects the area from the ribs to the pelvis. Thus you can move, "pushing" if you have to, but will not feel any pain.

Sources: *AMA Drug Evaluations,* 5th ed. (American Medical Association, 1983); Gilman, Alfred Goodman; Goodman, Louis S.; Gilman, Alfred, *The Pharmacological Basis of Therapeutics,* 6th ed. (Macmillan, 1980); Shnider, Sol M. "Choice of anesthesia for labor and delivery," *Obstetrics & Gynecology* (supplement), November 1981.

entire delivery, so it is important to discuss the alternatives with your doctor.

Among the drugs used during labor and delivery are local anesthetics, inhalation anesthetics and intravenous anesthetics.

Local anesthetics such as *bipivucaine, lidocaine* and *mepivicaine* allow a woman to stay awake and participate in the delivery of her baby. These drugs won't interfere with contractions, but they may affect the baby 's heartbeat and breathing. And, in 1983, after a number of women who had been given high concentrations of bipivucaine during delivery died of cardiac arrest, the FDA banned the use of high-concentration epidural injections of bipivucaine during labor and delivery. Questions about the safety and effectiveness of low-concentration bipivucaine remain to be answered.

Inhalation anesthetics. There are two ways to use these gases and volatile (fast-evaporating) liquids during labor. They can be inhaled in small doses from time to time for a momentary escape from pain, or, in higher concentrations, they can be used to produce general anesthesia (loss of consciousness), which is rarely, if ever, used in a normal, uncomplicated vaginal delivery.

All inhalation anesthetics can slow down heartbeat and respiration in mother and newborn. *Nitrous oxide,* a light anesthetic, is frequently used for momentary relief during labor. Although it has been linked to miscarriage among women who were exposed to it at work while they were pregnant, it is considered safe during childbirth. Low concentrations of *enflurane* and *methoxyflurane* will also provide relief without slowing down labor. At higher concentrations, however, enflurane can interfere with the uterus's ability to contract and may cause hemorrhage after the baby is born because it can keep your uterus from responding to the ergot or oxytocin used to make it contract once the placenta has been delivered. (See *Oxytocin,* p. 57; *Ergot,* p. 58.) *Halothane,* an otherwise popular inhalation anesthetic, can produce these effects even at low concentrations.

Intravenous anesthetics, such as the short-acting barbiturates *thiopental* (PENTOTHAL) and *methohexital* (BREVITAL), produce general anesthesia and are virtually never used in normal labor. They have very little effect on your contractions, but strongly depress respiration. *Meperidine* (DEMEROL) doesn't slow down labor or interfere with your uterus's ability to contract after the baby is born, but even moderate doses of this drug can cause a noticeable increase in the number of infants who have respiratory difficulty at birth.

Are the Drugs You Take while Breast-feeding Harmful for Your Baby?

Sometimes, they may be. Most of the drugs you use while you are breast-feeding will eventually show up in your breast milk. That goes for drugs you absorb through your skin as well as those you take by mouth or through injection. For example, women who use vaginal douches containing povidone-iodine may absorb the antiseptic through the walls of their vagina and pass it along to their nursing infants—who may begin to smell of iodine.

When you take a drug while you are nursing, how much will your infant get? In most cases, it is estimated that less than 2 percent of the amount you take will show up in your milk, but there are exceptions. If you use the antiasthma drug *theophylline,* for example, your milk may contain an amount equal to 10 percent of the dose you took. If you use the antimanic drug *lithium,* the concentration of lithium in your milk may approach 50 percent of the concentration of the drug in your body.

Here are some other drugs that may affect a baby when they show up in breast milk:

Analgesics. *Aspirin* is an anticoagulant. If used very often by a nursing mother, it may interfere with the normal clotting of her baby's blood. In one case, the baby of a nursing mother who took 200 mg. a day of the nonsteroidal anti-inflammatory analgesic *indomethacin* (INDOCIN) is reported to have suffered from convulsions. Repeated, large doses of *codeine* may be addictive for a nursing baby. The same is true of *morphine.*

Antibiotics. Babies can be sensitized to antibiotics they get in their mother's milk. In addition, the drugs can upset the normal bacterial balance in the infants' intestinal tracts. Babies whose mothers used *ampicillin* (AMCILL, OMNIPEN, PFIZERPEN-A, POLY-CILLIN) while nursing have suffered from diarrhea and the fungal infection candidiasis. Sulfa drugs in a nursing mother's milk can contribute to the development of kernicterus, a severe form of neonatal jaundice that can cause brain damage in the newborn. Tetracyclines can permanently discolor the baby's future teeth, and *trimethoprim,* which is most often given in combination with *sulfamethoxazole* as the urinary tract antiseptic BACTRIM or SEPTRA, may interfere with a newborn's ability to metabolize the vitamin folic acid.

Anticoagulants. The anticoagulants *phenindione* and *warfarin* (COUMADIN, PANWARFIN) have been reported to cause bleeding difficulties (including hemorrhage) in nursing infants.

Anticonvulsants. *Carbamazine* (TEGRETOL) is known to slow down the growing of nursing rats who get it in their mother's milk, but this effect has not been reported in human beings. *Phenytoin* (DILANTIN) has been reported to cause methemoglobinemia, a disorder of the hemoglobin (the red cells that carry oxygen to every part of the body) in babies nursed by mothers who were taking 400 milligrams a day.

Antihistamines. Not all antihistamines make people drowsy, but those that do may affect the nursing infant as well as the mother who takes them. Some antihistamines that make people sleepy are *brompheniramine maleate* (DIMETANE), *chlorpheniramine maleate* (CHLOR-TRIMETON, TELDRIN), *clemastine fumarate* (TAVIST), *dexchlorpheniramine maleate* (POLARAMINE), *promethazine HCl* (PHENERGEN) and *trimeprazine tartrate* (TEMANIL). Antihistamines may be hazardous for newborns and infants; always check with your doctor before using them while you are nursing.

Laxatives. If a nursing mother uses either *cascara* (MILK OF MAGNESIA-CASCARA, PERI-COLACE) or *danthron* (DOXIDAN, MODANE), her baby's bowel movements may be increased.

Oral contraceptives. The information on the effects of oral contraceptives on babies who get them in their mother's milk is contradictory, but they have been reported to cause gynecomastia (enlarged breasts) in a male infant and abnormal growth of vaginal tissue in a female infant.

Sedatives and tranquilizers. All the drugs that sedate you may also sedate your baby.

Steroid hormones. Corticosteroids *(cortisone, hydrocortisone)* can slow down your baby's growth and suppress her body's ability to produce a normal supply of her own.

Thyroid medication. The radioactive iodides used to treat hyperthyroidism (overactive thyroid) can show up in breast milk and may destroy the baby's thyroid gland or increase her chances of developing thyroid cancer later in life. Nonradioactive iodide drugs can stop the baby's thyroid gland from producing the thyroid hormones she needs and/or trigger goiter.

Tuberculosis drugs. The *isoniazid* (DOW-ISONIAZID, NYDRAZIA) taken by a nursing mother may damage her baby's liver.

Urinary antiseptics. *Nitrofuradantoin* (FURADANTIN, MACRODANTIN) in breast milk may cause the destruction of red blood cells in a nursing baby's body, a condition known as hemolytic anemia. (See also *Antibiotics,* p. 62.)

Vaginal antiseptics. *Povidone-iodine,* the antiseptic found in some vaginal douches and gels, can be absorbed through vaginal walls and excreted in breast milk. (See also *Thyroid medication,* above.)

Part IV

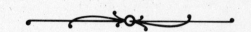

Medical Procedures

12. Do You Need Immunization?

There are two types of inoculations: those that require live viruses and those that use inactivated viruses or bacteria.

Live virus vaccines, as the name implies, give you a small dose of live virus which triggers a minor case of the illness so that your body begins to manufacture antibodies which will protect you in the future.

According to the Centers for Disease Control in Atlanta, it is usually safer to avoid all live-virus vaccines while you are pregnant because of the possibility that the virus may cross the placenta and infect your baby. However, the CDC does say that this rule may be waived if you face a serious threat of natural infection with yellow fever or polio (there is a killed-virus vaccine for polio, but the live-virus vaccine is considered more effective).

As for rubella vaccine, while it is always best to be cautious in dealing with rubella vaccine during pregnancy, you should be aware of the fact that there have never been any reports of a baby's developing congenital rubella (rubella acquired in the womb) when its mother was immunized while she was pregnant.

Killed-virus, killed-bacteria or toxoid vaccines use inactivated viruses, killed bacteria or anatoxins (toxins that have been treated to make them nontoxic although they still retain their ability to stimulate the production of antibodies in your system).

The CDC says that there is "no convincing evidence of risk to the fetus" from these vaccines. In fact, in 1983, researchers at the Magee-Women's Hospital and the University of Pittsburgh Medical School published the results of a five-year study showing that a fetus may actually be protected against tetanus when its mother is vaccinated while she is pregnant. Babies born to women who had been given tetanus antitoxin while pregnant had a higher level of antitetanus antibodies in their system for a full year after birth than babies whose mothers had not be inoculated.

Inoculations

Live-virus vaccines

BCG (immunization against tuberculosis)
Measles
Mumps
OPV (live-virus polio vaccine)
Rubella
Typhoid
Yellow fever
Varicella-zoster immune globulin (chicken pox, herpes zoster)

Killed-virus, killed-bacteria, toxoid vaccines

Cholera
Diphtheria
Influenza*
Pertussis
Plague
Tetanus

Sources: *AMA Drug Evaluations*, 5th ed. (American Medical Association, 1983); Centers for Disease Control, *Morbidity & Mortality Weekly Report*, Nov. 3, 1978, Nov. 2, 1979, Feb. 22, 1980, Feb. 29, 1980, Feb. 6, 1981, June 19, 1981; *The Medical Letter*, May 29, 1982.
* The CDC recommends this only during the 2nd and 3rd trimesters.

13. Has Your Doctor Suggested X-Rays?

Scientists have known for a long time that massive doses of radiation direction at the ovaries or testes can leave us sterile and that women who are exposed to large doses of radiation during cancer therapy may be temporarily infertile. But there is no evidence to suggest that the minimal doses of radiation that reach our ovaries or testes during an ordinary X-ray examination performed by a competent technician using well-maintained, modern equipment will affect our ability to produce a baby. What is worrisome, though, is whether the X-rays to which we are exposed before we conceive may damage sperm or egg so that the child they create will be born with birth defects.

Preconception X-rays and Birth Defects

Since all X-ray examinations expose us to ionizing radiation that can alter the genetic material inside living cells (including sperm and egg), it would seem logical to expect that preconception X-rays might cause changes that would show up in our future children. But, except for a few studies of Down's syndrome children showing that they seem to be more likely than other children to have had mothers or fathers who were exposed to repeated doses of radiation from preconception X-rays, there is no evidence to show that this is so. Why?

Perhaps the level of radiation we get from an ordinary X-ray examination is so low that it doesn't change the genetic material in sperm and egg, or perhaps the damage is so small that the cell can heal itself. People who espouse this argument point out that it takes an exposure to about at least 30,000 millirads (30 rads)* of ionizing

---

* Some researchers suggest that the amount of radiation needed to double the rate of mutation in human genes may be even higher.

radiation to double the rate of mutation in human genes, while an ordinary chest X-ray delivers about 1 millirad of radiation to the ovaries and none at all to the testes. (Other procedures may deliver significantly higher doses to the gonads, but nothing approaching 30,000 millirads.)

Perhaps the genetic damage the radiation causes in sperm or egg produces a recessive defect that won't show up in the first generation (your children) unless your mate also has a gene carrying the same recessive trait.

Perhaps the damage done by radiation from diagnostic X-rays alters genetic material in sperm or egg but doesn't produce visible defects in our children because the damaged sperm and egg are destroyed and never produce a baby.

Perhaps a badly damaged sperm or egg does combine with its healthy opposite to produce a baby, but we never see the damaged child because its defects are so severe that it is aborted spontaneously. One 1972 study, for example, appeared to suggest that women who miscarry may have a history of more preconception exposure to radiation from diagnostic X-rays than women who carry their babies successfully to term.

Finally, even if a damaged sperm or egg produces a damaged live-born child, we may still not see the effects, either because the damage is so slight or because in a population of several hundred million people exposed to literally hundreds of substances that may damage a developing fetus there is no way at all to link the baby's defects to a specific X-ray examination or series of X-ray examinations that took place before he was even conceived.

Protecting Your Reproductive Organs from Unnecessary Radiation

Because they, too, accept the possibility of radiation damage to ovaries, testes, sperm and eggs, radiologists usually try to avoid any unnecessary gonadal exposure during an X-ray examination. When you have one that involves an area near the gonads, the radiologist will use a protective shield if at all possible.

Obviously, this is easier to do with men than with women. Since the testes are outside the body and separate from the abdomen, shielding them won't interfere with a picture of the kidneys or bladder or intestines. (To further minimize the possibility of a radiation-damaged sperm's fertilizing a mature egg, many radiologists suggest your waiting three months after the X-ray examination be-

Estimated Average Radiation Dose to Ovaries or Testes during Some Common Diagnostic Medical X-Ray Procedures

Type of X-Ray Examination	Estimated Dose to the Ovaries* (in millirads)	Estimated Dose to the Testes* (in millirads)
Abdomen		
Kidney, ureter and bladder	221	97
Other abdomen studies	524	857
Back		
Cervical spine (neck)	—	—
Thoracic spine (between neck and abdomen)	11	3
Lumbar spine (between ribs and pelvis)	721	218
Chest	1	—
Dental (full mouth)	less than 10	less than 10
Gall bladder	78	—
Hip	124	600
Kidney (IVP)	588	207
Mammography	—	—
Pelvis	210	364
Shoulder	—	—
Skull	—	—
Upper GI series	171	1
Amount of radiation known to double the rate of mutation in human genes	30,000	

Source: *Effects of Ionizing Radiation on Developing Embryo and Fetus: A Review* (U.S. Department of Health and Human Services, Bureau of Radiological Health, August 1981); Laws, Priscilla, and Ralph Nader's Public Citizen Health Research Group, *The X-Ray Information Book* (Farrar, Straus and Giroux, 1983).

* These estimated doses, measured in millirads (a millirad is 1/1000th of a rad), are averages. The actual dose may vary considerably, depending on the quality of the X-ray machine and the skill of the operator. These figures (with the exception of the doses for dental X-rays and mammography) are exclusively for machines in the United States. Doses delivered by machines in other parts of the world may differ.

fore having unprotected intercourse that might result in your becoming pregnant.)

It is much more difficult to shield the ovaries from radiation during an X-ray examination of the lower trunk. All X-rays of the lower gastrointestinal tract, the kidneys, bladder, lower spine, hips, pelvis and thighs will involve some exposure of the ovaries.

Medical X-Rays During Pregnancy

If a woman is exposed to massive doses of ionizing radiation while pregnant, and the radiation strikes the uterus, there is a greater risk of her baby's growing more slowly in the womb or being deformed or dying before he is born. These effects were seen among pregnant women who lived through the atomic bomb blast at Hiroshima, where the levels of whole-body radiation were as high as 150,000 millirads in some places. The lowest whole-body dose of radiation known to produce specific birth defects is 10,000 millirads. Pregnant women at Hiroshima who were exposed to this level of radiation were more likely to deliver babies whose heads were smaller than normal, a condition known as microcephaly.

No ordinary diagnostic X-ray examination should produce anywhere near the dose of radiation women were exposed to at Hiroshima. In fact, according to the National Council on Radiation Protection and Measurements, less than 1 in every 1,000 radiographic examinations performed by competent technicians working with modern, well-maintained equipment produces more than 1,000 millirads, the level below which the probability of the baby's suffering a detectable birth defect is so slight that the benefits of the examination are generally considered to outweigh its possible hazards.

**Estimated Radiation Dose to Fetus during
Several Common Diagnostic
X-Ray Examinations Early in Pregnancy**

Type of X-Ray	Range of Estimated Dose to Fetus*
Abdomen (kidney, ureter and bladder)	50–700
Fetography	650
Gastrointestinal	
Upper GI series	5–110
Lower GI series	60–800
Gallbladder	1–20
Hip	30–470
Kidney (IVP)	50–480
Pelvis	60–280
Spine (between ribs and pelvis)	150–870

Source: *Effects of Ionizing Radiation on Developing Embryo and Fetus: A Review* (U.S. Department of Health and Human Services, Bureau of Radiological Health, August 1981).
* These estimated doses, measured in millirads (a millirad is 1/1000th of a rad), vary depending on the quality (and modernity) of the X-ray machine, as well as the skill of the person operating it. These ranges are for machines in the United States. X-ray machines in other parts of the world may well give different doses of radiation to the mother and the fetus for the same X-ray examination.

Does that mean there's no reason to worry about the effects your X-ray examination may have on your fetus? Not necessarily. While low-level radiation from diagnostic X-rays may not produce gross malformations or other detectible damage to your baby, the research in this area is just not far enough advanced to be able to say with certainty that there may not be subtle damage, such as changes in nerve cells, that no one can measure.

Protecting the Fetus from Unneccessary Radiation

If you must have an X-ray examination when you are (or might be) pregnant, the Public Health Service, an arm of the U.S. Department of Health and Human Services, has a number of suggested guidelines to help you and your doctor avoid exposing the baby you may be carrying to any unnecessary radiation:

If you are pregnant, let your doctor or X-ray technician know. It sound obvious, but the truth is that we sometimes forget to volunteer this information, perhaps because we assume that the doctor or technician already knows. It's much safer to assume that *nobody* knows, and to tell each new physician or technician you encounter.

Don't just assume you couldn't possibly be pregnant. Using The Pill or having an IUD in place is no guarantee that you have not conceived. Neither is the fact that your partner has had a vasectomy (for a short time after the operation or when the procedure has been botched, impregnation can occur). Even "infertile" couples have been known to conceive unexpectedly. Don't guess: ask your doctor or X-ray technician to evaluate your situation.

If it is at all possible that you might be pregnant, ask if the examination can be scheduled for a time when pregnancy is least likely. Although women have been known to conceive during their menstrual periods or during the ten days immediately following the start of the period, these are times when pregnancy is least likely to occur.

Have your X-ray examination done at a modern center, with trained technicians and up-to-date, well-maintained equipment. The risk of unnecessary radiation exposure during an X-ray examination rises if the technician is not well-trained or the machinery not in good working order.

If the examination is an emergency procedure, ignore all the previous rules and follow your doctor's advice.

How Radioactive Medicines and Radiation Therapy May Affect Your Baby

Large doses of radioactive iodine (which collect in the thyroid) are sometimes used to destroy an overactive gland. This treatment is not used after the sixth week of pregnancy because the radioactive iodine can destroy the fetus's thyroid as well as its mother's.

The effects of radiation therapy for cancer depend to a large extent on the strength of the dose, the frequency of the exposure and the site of the cancer. There have been reports linking radiation therapy during pregnancy to mental retardation, low birthweight, microcephaly (a smaller-than-normal head) and other malformations, particularly when the treatment took place between the third and twentieth weeks of pregnancy. But there have also been reports of healthy babies born to women who had massive doses of radiation therapy while they were pregnant.

14. Have You Had An Abortion?

There are two kinds of abortions, those that are induced medically and those that occur spontaneously.

A spontaneous abortion, also known as miscarriage, may be a signal that the fetus was simply not developing properly. Repeated miscarriage may be caused by chromosomal abnormalities; women who have a history of more than one miscarriage are often advised to consult with a genetic counselor because the same chromosomal abnormalities that cause the miscarriages may cause mongolism or other birth defects in a baby carried to term.

According to the results of a five-year study from the March of Dimes Birth Defects Foundation, women who have had two or more medically induced abortions (the procedure used to end an unsafe or unwanted pregnancy) have a higher risk of spontaneous abortion in the next pregnancy, but neither the March of Dimes report nor any of the other studies of the effects of induced abortion on fertility has shown any rise in the incidence of birth defects among babies born to women who had a history of induced abortions. Nor does induced abortion appear to lower fertility. In a study of more than 3,000 women at three different hospitals and clinics in Boston, a team of Harvard researchers found that the rate of subsequent pregnancy was actually higher among women who had had three or more abortions than among women who had had only one. One of the researchers, delivering the report to a meeting of the Association of Planned Parenthood Professionals in December 1982, suggested that the women who resorted to multiple induced abortions may have done so because they were more fertile than other women and more likely to fail to prevent pregnancy with contraception.

15. Where Will You Have Your Baby?

Home Birth vs. Birthing Center vs. Hospital Delivery

In the last few years, many women have begun to look for an alternative to what they perceive to be the impersonal, demeaning and sometimes dangerous experience of hospital delivery. The result has been an increase in home deliveries and the creation of "birthing centers," free-standing facilities where you can deliver your baby in an atmosphere warmer and more congenial than many hospitals can offer. In response, some hospitals have created "birthing rooms," cheerily decorated and less formal than a delivery room, but with a hospital staff in attendance.

The Advantages and Disadvantages of Home Birth. The primary advantage of home birth is psychological. With your family and perhaps your friends around you, birth is more likely to be the intensely personal and satisfying experience you want it to be. And so long as the delivery proceeds without any complications, having a baby at home gives you the best chance of controlling what's happening to you. There will be no predelivery enema or pubic shave unless you want it, and certainly no IV or anesthetics. On the other hand, if any problems arise, the disadvantages of home birth can be devastating. All deliveries carry at least the possibility of an unexpected hemorrhage. If that happens or if the baby has any problems at birth, the time spent getting to the nearest hospital could literally spell the difference between life and death.

The Advantages and Disadvantages of Birthing Centers. Birthing centers attempt to combine a warm and personal atmosphere with a professional approach to childbirth. Your care at the center begins well before delivery. The centers, which are independent but maintain an association with obstetricians and hospitals, will refer any woman whose pregnancy is considered high-risk to a doctor or hospital that can provide more sophisticated care. As with home delivery, birthing centers can provide a more congenial atmosphere than a hospital but may not be adequate in case of an emergency. The true measure of a birthing center's safety, therefore, lies in its ability to predict with accuracy which patients it should *not* treat.

The Advantages and Disadvantages of Hospital Delivery. Depending on the institution, the people in it, and your own doctor, having your baby in a hospital can be either warm and cooperative or cold, impersonal and miserable, just the sort of thing that sent women like you out looking for alternatives in the first place. When you deliver at home or in a birthing center, you get to make important decisions about how things will proceed, but entering a hospital generally means surrendering to a bureaucracy. This loss of control can be stressful even in the best of circumstances. During delivery, it can tighten your muscles and make your job that much more difficult. You may be able to alleviate the problem somewhat by discussing procedures completely with your obstetrician before you go into the hospital, but there is no guarantee that everything will go the way you want it to once you are actually there. To balance this well-known, frustrating aspect of hospital delivery, there is this saving grace: for a woman who faces a high-risk delivery or whose "normal" delivery suddenly turns into an emergency, the hospital offers the best chance for a safe outcome. (NOTE: Community hospitals often do not have the facilities to deal with high-risk pregnancy and delivery and may refer you to a major regional or teaching center where more sophisticated care is available.)

Obstetrical Procedures

Although it's sometimes difficult to do, it's really sensible to come to a discussion of obstetrical procedures with the same open mind you bring to a discussion of obstetrical drugs. No one disputes the fact that some of these procedures are intrusive and uncomfortable, probably unnecessary and possibly dangerous for mother and baby. But others are vital. They may spell the difference between success and failure in a difficult delivery.

Cesarean delivery. Cesareans now account for more than 15 percent of the deliveries each year in the United States. A cesarean is considered medically justifiable when used to hasten the birth of a baby who may be experiencing distress inside his mother's womb or to avoid the stress of abnormally prolonged labor on both mother and child. Every patient considered for a cesarean must be evaluated individually, but these are some of the situations in which your doctor may believe a cesarean is needed:

- if the placenta has moved from its normal position at the top of the uterus and is lying across the exit from the uterus to the cervix, a condition known as *placenta praevia* ("placenta first"); allowing labor to continue might lead to rupture of the placenta
- if you have hypertension, pre-eclampsia, diabetes, kidney disease or any other chronic condition that may put your baby at risk if the pregnancy is allowed to continue to the "normal" delivery date
- if you have a chronic condition that might cause abnormally prolonged labor, increasing the chances that your baby may be deprived of oxygen
- if you have an active herpes infection
- if your baby is in a breech position and cannot be delivered vaginally; in one study of births in New York City between 1970 and 1978, there was no consistent difference in survival rates among breech babies born by cesarean vs. those born vaginally so long as the baby weighed less than five pounds, but breech babies weighing more than five pounds were five times more likely to live if delivered by cesarean
- if your baby's head is too large to pass through your pelvic arch without injuring either one of you

The baby does face risks during cesarean delivery. For example, there is a higher incidence of neonatal respiratory distress among babies delivered by cesarean than among those delivered vaginally, but some people think that this may simply be because more high-risk infants are delivered by cesarean.

Healthy babies delivered by cesarean may face an increased risk of iatrogenic prematurity (prematurity caused by the doctor) if the obstetrician decides to hasten the birth of an otherwise perfect baby whose lungs are not mature enough to keep him alive outside his mother's body. To avoid this, the doctor will take a sample of the amniotic fluid before scheduling a cesarean. The fluid contains two fats, lecithin (made in the baby's lungs) and sphingomyelin (made in his skin). At the beginning of pregnancy, the ratio of lecithin to sphingomyelin in the amniotic fluid is 1:1, but as birth draws near, there is a spurt in lecithin production that signals a spurt in lung development. When the baby is ready to be born, there will be about twice as much lecithin as sphingomyelin in the amniotic fluid.

The anesthesia used for cesarean delivery is usually stronger than what is given for a vaginal delivery. It depresses the baby's respiration as well as the mother's, but, according to the National Institutes of Health Consensus Development Conference on Cesarean Birth, there still isn't enough information or research to say exactly what effects the stronger anesthetic will have on the baby's eventual physical and intellectual development.

Mothers, too, may have some problems. Women who deliver by cesarean are two to four times more likely to die during childbirth than women who deliver vaginally. To some extent, this reflects the fact that many of these women are ill before they get to the delivery room. Nonetheless, a cesarean is major surgery. It carries all the risks of infection or anesthesia-related complications we associate with any other abdominal surgery.

If you have one cesarean delivery, will you be able to deliver your next baby vaginally? Perhaps. Many women do, but a lot depends on your own physiology and the reason you had the cesarean in the first place. Clearly, this is one of those decisions that has to be made woman by woman, one at a time.

Other obstetrical procedures. It was once standard obstetrical practice to give laboring women an enema to empty the lower colon and reduce the contamination that can occur naturally when a baby is being born. Now, however, most doctors recognize what most women always knew, that an enema can increase the intensity of natural contractions, sometimes making them so strong that you cannot control them and may need anesthesia you could otherwise have avoided. As a result, the enema before delivery is becoming an increasingly rare event.

Another standard obstetrical procedure is the insertion of an intravenous needle in your hand or arm when labor begins. Because it is impossible to guarantee that labor will proceed without problems from start to finish, it is extremely valuable to have an IV in place in case you need drugs or a blood transfusion in a hurry. A second reason for insertion of the IV is to provide nutrients and liquids during labor. Most obstretricians prefer not to have you eat once labor begins because they believe that it may nauseate you or pose the risk of your aspirating food if you suddenly need general anesthesia during delivery. On the other hand, some women's groups believe that eating lightly while you are in labor can actually prevent nausea and may help you relax.

Whether or not to shave the pubic area before a vaginal delivery has become a matter of legitimate controversy. This procedure, which some women find embarrassing or demeaning, is done ostensibly to prevent infection, but there is no medical evidence to show that it does. In fact, some studies have shown that shaving the skin appears to increase your chances of infection. As a result, in many hospitals shaving is no longer an absolute standard during vaginal delivery. However, if your obstetrician believes that an episiotomy is necessary, she will probably have to shave that area so as to have a clear field for the incision.

The idea of a forceps delivery raises strong emotions in both doctor and patient. There is no doubt that many babies have been injured by the indiscriminate use of forceps, particularly high forceps that reach far up into the birth canal and must pull the baby down a long distance at what may be a contorted angle. But, like cesarean delivery, forceps delivery may be used to rescue a baby in respiratory distress or to shorten an unusually long labor.

As an obstetrical tool, forceps may eventually yield entirely to a new instrument, the silastic (for *sil*icone *elast*omer) cup. This is a soft plastic vacuum cup which fits onto the baby's head and helps the obstetrician ease the infant's passage down the birth canal. The cup is not yet in general use, but an eight-month study at the University of Texas Medical School at San Antonio showed that it was less likely than forceps to injure either mother or child. One feature which makes the cup especially safe for the baby is the fact that it will slip off the infant's head if it is not applied properly or if a great deal of force is required to pull the baby down the birth canal (in which case, the doctor may opt for a cesarean instead of forcing the baby out into the world).

Part V

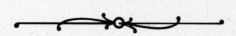

Nutrition

16. What Do You Eat and Drink?

Food and Beverages as Aphrodisiacs

Although folk medicine credits many foods with aphrodisiac qualities, the truth is that there is no single, special food or drink that will guarantee either potency or fertility. Why, then, do so many foods have that special reputation? In *Consuming Passions,* a book devoted to the anthropological aspects of eating, authors Peter Farb and George Armelagos suggested a few answers.

Sometimes it is because the supposed aphrodisiac is actually a stimulant that may improve our mood and our attitude toward a particular romantic encounter. Coffee and tea, which contain caffeine, may fall into this category. Other "aphrodisiacs" are irritants that produce an uncomfortable sensation in the urinary tract which some people may interpret as a prelude to arousal. The oil in pepper can do this; so can curries and other strong spices or hot spicy foods.

Occasionally, foods may seem to have sexual magic because they look like the genitalia or are somehow related to reproduction. Bananas, asparagus, and carrots fit neatly into the first group; caviar and roe (fish eggs), into the latter.

And then there are the foods whose specialness comes from the fact that they are new. Two examples, which may seem strange to us today, are tomatoes (love apples) and potatoes, once new, strange and wonderful to the Europeans.

Finally, there are the foods with a tenuous but absolutely scientific link to reproduction. Oysters are a good example. They are rich in zinc, which is essential for sperm production, but it's a good bet that their folk reputation comes from their "strangeness," since you can get plenty of zinc from meat or plant foods.

Calories Count at Every Stage

Exactly how many calories does your body need each day? According to the National Research Council, a normal, healthy adult woman who isn't pregnant or nursing needs between 10 and 25 calories a day for each pound of body weight. A normal, healthy adult man needs a little more, about 15–27 calories a day for each pound of body weight. The range is meant to account for a number of variables, including how active you are and how your own individual metabolism runs.

What if your diet has enough calories but is missing some important nutrients? Simply put, any diet that relies on one food or one group of foods to the exclusion (or near-exclusion) of all others can lead to malnutrition that, in turn, may interfere with ovulation or libido.

Sometimes exclusionary diets are easy to spot (an all-meat

**Daily Calorie Allowances
for Normal, Healthy Adult Men and Women**

Age	Height/ Weight*	Energy (calorie) Requirements
Women†		
15–18	5'4" 120 lbs.	1,200–3,000
19–22	5'4" 120 lbs.	1,700–2,500
23–50	5'4" 120 lbs.	1,600–2,400
Men		
15–18	5'9" 145 lbs.	2,100–3,900
19–22	5'10" 154 lbs.	2,500–3,300
23–50	5'10" 154 lbs.	2,300–3,100

Source: *Recommended Dietary Allowances* (National Research Council, 1980).
* Mean heights and weights. (Mean = the point in the middle.)
† Neither pregnant nor nursing.

high-protein diet, for example, or a grapefruit diet), but sometimes they aren't. Vegetarianism, which includes protein foods like cheese, milk and eggs, is a healthful way of life, but a vegan diet (which differs from vegetarianism in that it avoids *all* animal foods, including milk, cheese and eggs) may be lacking several nutrients, including vitamin B_{12}.

The best rule is to avoid all fad diets. They just don't have what it takes to help you maintain a healthy reproductive life.

Getting enough calories during pregnancy. Pregnancy is not the time to go on a reducing diet. In fact, even if you are slightly over-weight when you become pregnant, your doctor will expect you to gain weight while you are carrying the baby because if you do not get the extra calories you need, your baby may not get the energy it needs to maintain normal growth inside the womb.

It's been estimated that it takes about 80,000 extra calories—over and above your "normal" diet—to meet all the demands of a nine-month pregnancy. That works out to about 300 extra calories a day. While the figure has swung back and forth over the years, today the recommended weight gain during pregnancy is usually put at 25–30 pounds; a woman who fails to gain at least 10 pounds during her first trimester may have a higher risk of giving birth to a low-birthweight infant.

All these figures apply to healthy, adult women. Teenagers who aren't fully grown when they become pregnant may need to add even more calories and gain even more weight. In one study of adolescent weight gain, researchers found that most young girls gain an average of 35 pounds of fatty tissue at puberty. Interestingly enough, this weight gain is equal to about 120,000 calories, the amount needed to sustain a nine-month pregnancy and provide an extra cushion for three months spent nursing a newborn baby. Nature is *very* practical.

Calories after delivery. After the baby is born, some women cut back on calories in an attempt to lose weight quickly. But a woman who is breast-feeding will need more food energy, not less. It takes about 800 extra calories every day to produce enough milk to feed a healthy infant without endangering the mother's own nutritional status. The fat stored during pregnancy can give a nursing mother some of the extra calories she needs, but she will still need to consume about 500 calories more each day than she did before she was pregnant. The stored fat is normally depleted after about three months, so a woman who nurses longer than that will need to increase her calorie consumption. Women who are breast-feeding more than one infant or who were underweight before or during pregnancy will also need more than 500 extra calories every day while nursing.

Special Diets and Special Cautions

Vegetarian diets. During pregnancy, a vegetarian diet that includes milk, cheese and eggs usually provides an adequate supply of all the essential vitamins and minerals except iron, which is hard to get without meat or an iron supplement. The vegetarian diet has the benefit of being high in fiber, which means that it may help to alleviate constipation. However, a high-fiber diet is also high in phytates, substances in cereals and plant food that can interfere with your body's absorption of zinc, copper and some other nutrients.

A vegan diet may not provide enough calcium for a pregnant woman. It may also be deficient in the B vitamins and in vitamin D. Since you need vitamin D to absorb and hold calcium in your bones, without it you may develop osteomalacia, an adult vitamin-D deficiency disease often seen in pregnant women in Asia and India who follow a vegan diet. To avoid osteomalacia, many vegans use vitamin D–enriched soy milk. Vegetarian diets that rely on cooked vegetables, rather than fresh, raw ones, may be low in folic acid.

One problem common to all vegetarian diets is that they are lower in calories than diets containing meat. (Vegan diets are lower in calories than vegetarian diets.) Vegetarian women often weigh less than women who eat meat. If they are very thin, they may have trouble becoming pregnant. Once pregnant, they must be careful to eat enough food to provide all the calories required for a successful pregnancy. This can be hard, particularly for adolescent vegetarians.

Finally, vegans and vegetarians may have only marginal reserves of some essential nutrients. Producing milk for a nursing infant can deplete these reserves, so it's important for nursing women who follow these diets to be certain that they are getting all the nutrients they need to meet the needs of two people, a mother *and* her child.

"Health food" diets. Some people who follow a "health food" diet are vegetarians; others will eat meat, chicken and fish. What both groups have in common is the desire to avoid foods that have been processed or that contain synthetic additives. People on "health food" diets also tend to emphasize vitamin and mineral supplements.

In practice, this usually means opting for a diet rich in fresh fruits and vegetables grown with "natural" fertilizers, whole grains, molasses or honey or brown sugar instead of refined white sugar, meat or chicken from animals raised on feed free of hormones or antibiotics, and vitamin and mineral supplements made without starches, sugar or artificial colors and flavors.

While a health food diet may be expensive, as long as it is varied, it is usually wholesome and nutritious. Just about the only problem it may pose for a pregnant woman is that a strong reliance on vitamins and minerals may lead to the consumption of very large doses of some nutrients that can cross the placenta and may endanger the fetus or show up in a nursing mother's milk.

Foods That May Contain Hazardous Contaminants

Some common foods may contain contaminants that may be harmful to the fetus.

Raw meat or meat that has not been thoroughly cooked. Such meat may contain *T. gondii,* a small parasite said to look something like a banana. *T. gondii* is the organism that causes toxoplasmosis, an infection that is extremely dangerous for the fetus. Nearly 35 percent of the women who get toxoplasmosis while they are pregnant pass it on to the fetus. Then the chances of giving birth to a baby with congenital toxoplasmosis depend to a great extent on when the parasite was picked up. The chances of the baby's becoming infected in the womb rise from 17 percent if one gets toxoplasmosis during the first trimester of pregnancy to 65 percent if it is picked up during the last three months. About 70 percent of the babies born with toxoplasmosis will show no symptoms at all when they are born. One in 10 will have some kind of eye damage, and 20 percent will have jaundice or anemia or fever or a rash or a blood disorder or be mentally retarded. However, even those who show no symptoms at birth may eventually lose their sight or be mentally retarded or die.

Organ foods. The liver is a "detoxifying" organ that helps to remove contaminants from the blood. As a result, many contaminants in animal feed—hormones, pesticides, antibiotics—end up in beef, calf, pork and chicken liver, and some experts advise against a pregnant woman's eating liver or pâtés because of the risk of exposing the fetus to these potentially harmful substances.

Fish. Like cattle and poultry, fish may be contaminated with substances in their environment and pass the contamination on to us. Some common environmental contaminants in fish are methylmercury, dioxins and polychlorinated biphenyls (PCBs).

Methylmercury is a waste product sometimes found in the water near plants where mercury is used in the manufacture of batteries, electrical parts, pharmaceuticals and pesticides. Mercury is a central nervous system poison that can cause cerebral palsy and microcephaly (an abnormally small head) in babies born to women who eat fish contaminated with the toxic metal while they are pregnant. The most famous case of fetal mercury poisoning occurred during the early 1960s in Minimata, Japan, where pregnant women had eaten fish contaminated with mercury waste from a nearby chemical plant.

In some parts of the United States, fish have also been contaminated with dioxins and PCBs. One dioxin, TCDD (2,3,7,8-tetra-chlorodibenzo-p-dioxin), is the contaminant in "Agent Orange." Small amounts of TCDD fed to pregnant laboratory rats may kill the fetuses.

To avoid exposure to dioxins and PCBs in the waters of the Great Lakes and the Hudson River, pregnant women are usually advised to avoid all large fish, including salmon, lake trout, rainbow trout, brown trout, smallmouth bass and eels. The larger the fish, the more likely it is to contain hazardous amounts of any contaminants in the water in which it swims.

Canned foods. In 1983, the Food and Drug Administration's Bureau of Foods validated one long-standing bit of folk wisdom when it officially advised consumers to remove canned food from the can as soon as it is opened. The reason is simple. Two-thirds of the more than 30 billion cans of food sold in this country every year are sealed with lead solder. When the can is opened, oxygen mixes with the food inside, making it more likely that lead will be drawn out of the solder. (Refrigerating the opened can will not prevent lead contamination of the food.)

This problem is most acute with acid foods such as fruit or fruit juices. In one case cited by the FDA, lead levels as high as 830 micrograms per serving were discovered in a can of orange juice that had been open for several days. According to the FDA, that is eight times the permissible safe maximum daily intake. In human beings, lead poisoning during pregnancy has been linked to spontaneous abortion and stillbirth, as well as malformations of the fetus's central nervous system.

Note that this is one of those news stories you must read very carefully. Canned foods can be a convenient source of nutritious food for a varied diet, so it is important to remember that current information links the problem of lead contamination *only* to foods that have been left standing in an opened can whose seams are sealed with lead solder.

Is the Alcohol You Drink a Hazard?

Alcohol and Sex. Alcoholic beverages have always been regarded as aphrodisiacs, pleasant and sophisticated accompaniments to a romantic encounter. It is true that small or moderate amounts of alcohol can relax inhibitions and tensions, sometimes making it easier to deal with sexual activity, but large amounts of alcohol can make it difficult for both men and women to respond sexually. Men who drink too much may not be able to achieve or maintain an erection. Male alcoholics may be both impotent and sterile, and the liver damage that often goes along with alcoholism may lead to a hormonal imbalance (too much estrogen, too little testosterone) that results in feminization characterized by gynecomastia (enlarged breasts). Women who drink too much may temporarily lose the ability to control vaginal muscle pressure.

Alcohol beverages may pose particular problems for adolescents. In 1981, researchers at the University of Illinois in Chicago reported that regular doses of ethanol, the alcohol in beer, wine and spirits, appeared to delay sexual maturity in adolescent mice. To date, there has not been any follow-up study of adolescent boys and girls who drink.

Fetal Alcohol Syndrome. Early in the 1970s, a team of researchers at the University of Washington in Seattle recognized that babies born to alcoholic women who continued to drink heavily (six drinks a day or more) while they were pregnant often showed a specific pattern of birth defects, including low birthweight, facial malformations, heart defects, and mental retardation. The researchers called this group of defects "fetal alcohol syndrome."

Ever since then, the question of exactly how much alcohol will trigger fetal alcohol syndrome has been a matter of heated debate. In 1983, a study reported in *Obstetrics & Gynecology,* the journal of the American College of Obstetricians and Gynecologists, attempted to clarify the issues by defining levels of consumption and matching them up with evidence of birth defects.

The Boston University scientists who wrote the article began by defining one drink as the amount of beer, wine or spirits that delivers 0.5 ounces of absolute alcohol: 12 ounces of 8-proof beer, 4 ounces of 24-proof wine, and 1.2 ounces of 80-proof distilled spirits. (NOTE: "Proof" is calculated by doubling the percentage of alcohol in the beverage. For example, wine that is marked "12 percent alcohol by volume" is 24 proof.)

Then they defined categories of drinkers. A "heavy drinker" would be a person who takes at least 5 drinks on some occasions and always has at least 45 drinks a month. A "rare drinker" would be someone who doesn't drink at all or who takes a drink less often than once a month and who never has 5 drinks on any one occasion.

A "moderate drinker" would be someone whose consumption pattern is somewhere in between these two extremes.

Using these criteria and eliminating defects that could be pinned on smoking, drugs, prepregnancy weight and a number of other variables, the researchers said that their observation of 469 mother/infant pairs at Boston City Hospital seemed to show that women who drank heavily while they were pregnant had a significantly higher chance of giving birth to a baby with fetal alcohol syndrome. They added that they had found no such link between alcohol and birth defects in babies born to women who were rare or moderate drinkers although two subsequent studies at Columbia University have suggested that women who drink very little (one drink a week) may have an increased risk of miscarriage.

Knowing *what* happens is only half the story. Knowing *how* it happens is the other half. In 1982, a group of medical researchers at Vanderbilt University Medical Center in Nashville, who were studying fetal alcohol syndrome, fed alcohol to pregnant rats and discovered that when the mother drinks, the fetus develops a zinc deficiency. Zinc is an essential nutrient. It makes protein synthesis possible and without an adequate supply, the fetus will not grow properly. Hence, fetal alcohol syndrome. The researchers found that even a single dose of alcohol measurably decreased the amount of zinc the fetus received across the placenta. However, single doses didn't cause any permanent damage (which supports the Boston researchers' conclusion that rare drinking isn't linked to fetal damage). In a follow-up study in 1983, the Vanderbilt doctors tried to correct the fetal zinc deficiencies by giving pregnant rats zinc supplements along with their daily doses of alcohol. It did not work. Even with the mothers getting supplements, the fetuses did not get enough zinc.

Because of the uncertainty regarding the precise dose of beverage alcohol that may be hazardous during pregnancy, some health organizations, including the American Medical Association and the March Of Dimes Birth Defects Foundation, suggest that abstinence may be the only safe course, a position currently endorsed by the Surgeon General of the United States. Others, such as the American College of Obstetricians and Gynecologists, believe that either moderation *or* abstinence may be prudent. There will certainly be more to come on this story.

What breast-feeding mothers need to know about alcohol. When you drink beer, wine, spirits or other alcohol beverages, most of the alcohol that is not actually oxidized inside your body is eliminated through your kidneys or lungs. Small amounts may show up in sweat, tears, saliva or other body secretions, including breast milk. If you drink large amounts of alcohol while you are nursing, your infant may feel the effects. For example, one infant whose mother had consumed about five ounces of port wine over a 24-hour period began to show symptoms of intoxication.

Is the Coffee You Drink While You Are Pregnant a Problem for Your Baby?

In some studies of pregnant animals, very high doses of caffeine (equivalent to 25 or more cups of coffee a day) have been linked to a variety of fetal malformations, and two studies of human beings have appeared to show a higher incidence of birth defects among babies born to women who had taken more than 8 cups of coffee a day while they were pregnant. Later studies, however, seem to exonerate moderate amounts of caffeine. In January 1982, a Harvard University research team that had put together case histories for 12,205 women who had given birth at Boston's Brigham and Women's Hospital reported in the *New England Journal of Medicine* that they had found no correlation between drinking coffee while pregnant and giving birth prematurely or giving birth to a low-birthweight infant. Two months later, researchers at Boston University reported in the *Journal of the American Medical Association* that they had been unable to find any link between coffee-drinking during pregnancy and six specific birth defects (inguinal hernia, cleft lip with or without cleft palate, cleft palate alone, pyloric stenosis [a closure of the opening from the stomach into the intestines], and spina bifida).

Some Foods That May Show Up in Breast Milk

The garlic, onions, legumes, cabbage and fresh fruit (melons, rhubarb, peaches and so forth) that you eat while you are nursing may make your infant colicky if she is sensitive to them; not all nursing babies are.

The milk you drink may also affect your baby. In one Swedish study of 19 colicky infants, 13 recovered promptly when their mothers stopped drinking cow's milk.

Do you drink coffee, tea or soft drinks? If so, some of the caffeine you are consuming will be excreted in your milk.

Chocolate, which contains a little caffeine in addition to the muscle stimulant theobromine, is on nearly everybody's list of foods to avoid while nursing. However, a recent (1981) study at the Milton S. Hershey Medical Center of the Pennsylvania State University of Medicine suggests that when a nursing mother eats a normal amount of chocolate (about one ordinary bar), the amount of caffeine and theobromine her baby gets is so small as to be insignificant.

17. Are There Harmful Additives in Your Food

During the 1960s, when it became evident that some of the chemicals we had been adding routinely to our food might be carcinogenic, the Food and Drug Administration, together with the companies that make and market these additives, initiated an ambitious testing program to find out whether or not our food additives were safe.

As the testing went along, information about how food additives may affect reproduction began to emerge. Today, scientists are able to talk about three broad categories of additives: those that have not yet been tested on pregnant animals, those that have been tested on pregnant animals and seem to be safe, and those that have been tested on pregnant animals and seem to be potentially dangerous.

It is important to remember, though, that these categories are still *very* elastic. As science becomes more sophisticated, additives may move from one category into another. Much of what you will read here and in your daily newspaper, therefore, must still be considered preliminary, one step along the way to an eventual certainty.

Additives That Have Not Yet Been Tested on Pregnant Animals

Although years of experience may suggest that some of these additives are safe for use by pregnant animals and human beings, lack of scientific evidence means that there simply is no way to be certain. As the FDA tests continue, this list can be expected to shrink dramatically.

Some Food Additives That
Have Not Yet Been Tested on Pregnant Animals

Ammonium alginate	Thickener
Ammonium carbonate	Leavening agent
Ammonium chloride	Dough conditioner
Ammonium hydroxide	Leavening agent
Ammonium sulfate	Dough conditioner
Calcium alginate	Thickener
Calcium sulfate	Dough conditioner
Caramel	Flavor, color
Cellulose derivatives	Thickeners
Choline bitartrate	Nutrient
Choline chloride	Nutrient
Cochineal	Color
Corn sweetener	Flavor
Dioctyl sodium sulfosuccinate	Surfactant
Glycerides (monoglycerides, diglycerides, monosodium diglycerides)	Emulsifiers
Glyceryl abietate	Plasticizer (texturizer)
Mannitol	Sweetener, anticaking agent
Potassium alginate	Thickener
Potassium sulfate	Nutrient
Smoke flavoring	Flavor
Sodium alginate	Thickener
Sodium sulfate	Nutrient
Sodium lauryl sulfate	Surfactant
Tumeric, tumeric oleoresin	Colors
Vanillin, ethyl vanillin	Flavors

Sources: Freydberg, Nicholas, and Gortner, Willis, *The Food Additives Book* (Bantam, 1982); Jacobson, Michael, *Eater's Digest* (Anchor Books, 1976); *Registry of Toxic Effects of Chemical Substances* (National Institute for Occupational Safety and Health, 1982); Winter, Ruth, *A Consumer's Dictionary of Food Additives* (Crown, 1978).

Additives That Have Been Tested on Pregnant Animals and Do Not Seem to Harm the Fetus

It is best to be very cautious about applying information from animal testing to human beings. Animals are different from people. Some chemicals that are safe for them aren't safe for us, and vice versa. In addition, the species chosen for the test can affect the outcome. One good example of this is the drug *thalidomide*. This sedative caused birth defects in thousands of children whose mothers took it while they were pregnant. However, thalidomide is much less likely to cause birth defects in rat and mice embryos than in rabbit, monkey and human embryos. The additives listed in the chart have been tested in pregnant animals and, to date, do not appear to affect the fetus or its mother in the amounts usually found in our food. To be safe, however, check with your own physician before using foods containing these additives.

Some Food Additives That Have Been Tested on Pregnant Animals and Do Not Seem to Harm the Fetus

Acetic acid	Preservative, flavor, acidifier
Adipic acid	Antioxidant, acidifier
Aluminum compounds	Firming agents, acidifiers
Azodicarbonamide	Dough conditioner
Benzoic acid	Preservative
Bromelain	Enzyme
Calcium chloride	Nutrient
Calcium gluconate	Buffer, firming agent
Citric acid and other citrates	Flavor enhancer, preservative
Cysteine	Antioxidant, dough conditioner
Disodium guanylate (GMP)	Flavor enhancer
Disodium inosinate (IMP)	Flavor enhancer
Ethyl formate	Flavor enhancer
Formic acid	Flavor enhancer
Glucono-delta-lactone	Acidifier, leavening agent
Glutamic acid	Flavor enhancer
Glycerin (glycerol)	Moisturizer, plasticizer
Hydrolyzed animal and vegetable proteins	Flavor enhancers
Lecithin (soy)	Emulsifier
Malic acid	Flavoring
Maltol	Flavor, flavor enhancer
Modified food starch	Thickener
MSG*	Flavor enhancer
Pectin	Gel
Phosphates, Phosphoric acid	Flavoring agents, emulsifiers, pH adjusters
Potassium bromate	Dough conditioner
Potassium chloride	Flavor enhancer, nutrient
Potassium hydroxide	Alkalizer (neutralizes acidity)

**Some Food Additives That Have Been Tested on Pregnant Animals
and Do Not Seem to Harm the Fetus (*cont.*)**

Propionic acid	Preservative, mold inhibitor
Polysorbate 60, polysorbate 80	Emulsifiers
Sodium benzoate	Preservative
Sorbic acid	Preservative, mold inhibitor
Sorbitan monostearate	Emulsifier
Sorbitol	Sweetener
Stannous chloride	Antioxidant
Tannic acid	Flavoring
Tartaric acid	Flavoring
Xanthan gum	Thickener, stabilizer, emulsifier

Sources: Freydberg, Nicholas; Gortner, Willis, *The Food Additives Book* (Bantam, 1982); Jacobson, Michael, *Eater's Digest* (Anchor Books, 1976); *Registry of Toxic Effects of Chemical Substances* (National Institute for Occupational Safety and Health, 1982); Winter, Ruth, *A Consumer's Dictionary of Food Additives* (Crown, 1978).
* MSG may be hazardous for newborns and infants.

Additives That Have Been Tested on Pregnant Animals and Appear to Be Harmful

In some cases, tests on laboratory animals have been able to pinpoint additives that may pose special problems for pregnant mice, rats, rabbits, monkeys and the like. Once again, it is best to be cautious in applying these results to people, although the ethical considerations that keep us from testing additives on human beings mean that these animal tests may be our only guide to possible hazards.

Agar-agar

A gel made from seaweed. When doses several thousand times the amount likely to be used by human beings were fed to pregnant mice, many more mice died than would ordinarily have been expected and there was a lowered birth rate among the ones who survived. This did not happen in any other species or when the amount of agar-agar given the mice was cut in half.

Alginates (alginic acid, ammonium, calcium, potassium, sodium, propylene glycol alginate)

Thickeners made from algae (seaweeds). One alginate, propylene glycol alginate, was linked to a rise in maternal and fetal deaths when doses more than 3,000 times the amount normally eaten by people were given to pregnant mice. To date, none of the other alginates have been tested on pregnant animals.

BHT and BHA

The evidence about butylated hydroxyanisole (BHA) and butylated hydroxytoluene (BHT) has been see-sawing back and forth for more than 25 years. In 1959, researchers reported that a diet that was 0.5 percent BHT caused pregnant rats to give birth to infants without eyes, but six years later, scientists working with BHA and BHT were unable to get the same results, even with much higher doses of the additives (which are antioxidants). Today, some experts believe that BHA and BHT are safe, while others say that they appear to stimulate the activity of steroid enzymes and thus may affect reproduction.

EDTA

In 1971, an article in *Science* magazine described tests in which large amounts of EDTA (ethylenediaminetetracetic acid) fed to pregnant rats were linked to cleft palate, brain and eye defects and skeletal deformities in their offspring. However, because the researchers were able to prevent these deformities by adding zinc to the pregnant rats' diets, they suggest that the effects may have been due to a zinc deficiency caused by the EDTA's "binding" the zinc the rats ate, making it unavailable for body use. (EDTA is used to bind metal contaminants, keeping them from causing color, flavor and texture changes in food.)

Guar gum

A thickener used to improve the way food tastes and feels in your mouth. When pregnant mice were given the gum in amounts more than 1,000 times what you would expect to find in a daily human diet, the death rate among the animals went up.

Quinine

As a drug, quinine is used to treat malaria. As a food additive, it is used to give that pleasantly bitter taste to tonic water, some "bitter-lemon" drinks, and some aperatifs. Taken during the first trimester of pregnancy, quinine may act as an abortifacient; it may also be linked to fetal malformation. During the nineteenth century, when quinine was used in an attempt to end unwanted pregnancies, women who took the drug but did not abort often gave birth to babies who were deaf. Quinine's ability to damage auditory nerves has been confirmed in modern animal research and suggested in some surveys of human infants. Although the amount of quinine in beverages is very small (approximately 80 milligrams per quart of quinine water and 20 milligrams per quart of bitter-lemon beverages) compared to the amount known to damage the fetus (600 mg.), many researchers suggest avoiding the risk entirely.

Sodium nitrite

Helps to protect foods against botulism. A potential carcinogen. While it has not been linked to birth defects, infants born to pregnant rats and guinea pigs who had been fed food and water containing 0.3–0.5 percent sodium nitrite grew more slowly and died more often than did infants born to control animals who had not gotten the sodium nitrite.

Food Additives and Fertility

There is very little hard information about how food additives affect fertility. In a few cases, however, tests on animals seem to suggest a *tenuous* connection between certain food additives and the reproductive system.

Brominated vegetable oils (BVO) are oils to which the element bromine has been added. Adding bromine makes the oil heavier so that it will not separate out of liquids with which it is mixed. BVOs are used as vehicles for flavoring agents in soft drinks and sweetened fruit drinks. When pigs were given doses of brominated sesame and soybean oils 2,500 times higher than those likely to be found in a human diet, the pigs' testicles began to shrivel.

Phenylmethyl cyclosiloxane is used to keep dry ingredients, like flour, from caking. In one study, phenylmethyl cyclosiloxane seemed to cause atrophied testicles and lowered sperm production in several species of animals, including monkeys.

Propyl gallate is an antioxidant, used to keep oil from turning rancid. Doses 25,000 times the amount normally found in a human diet reduced fertility in pregnant rats, but the problem disappeared when the dose was cut in half.

18. Do You Take Vitamin and Mineral Supplements?

Vitamins and minerals initiate and maintain the chemical action in living cells. While an adequate supply of these nutrients won't *guarantee* good health, a diet that delivers less than we need will almost certainly keep our bodies from working properly. Exactly what doses are right for each of us is a matter of some controversy, but the recommendations of the National Research Council do provide a basic, conservative guide.

Recommended Daily Dietary Allowance of Vitamins and Minerals for Women of Child-Bearing Age

Vitamin/ Mineral	15–18 years*	19–22 years	23+ years
Vitamin A	4,000 IU†	4,000 IU	4,000 IU
Vitamin D	400 IU	300 IU	200 IU
Vitamin E	12 IU‡	12 IU	12 IU
Vitamin C	60 mg.	60 mg.	60 mg.
Thiamin	1.1 mg.	1.1 mg.	1.0 mg
Riboflavin	1.3 mg.	1.3 mg.	1.2 mg.
Niacin	14 mg.	14 mg.	13 mg.
Vitamin B_6	2.0 mg	2.0 mg.	2.0 mg.
Folacin	400 mcg.	400 mcg.	400 mcg.
Vitamin B_{12}	3.0 mcg.	3.0 mcg.	3.0 mcg.
Calcium	1,200 mg.	800 mg.	800 mg.
Phosphorus	1,200 mg.	800 mg.	800 mg.
Magnesium	300 mg.	300 mg.	300 mg.
Iron	18 mg.	18 mg.	18 mg.§
Zinc	15 mg.	15 mg.	15 mg.
Iodine	150 mcg.	150 mcg.	150 mcg.

Recommended Daily Dietary Allowances of Vitamins and Minerals for Adult Men

Vitamin/ Mineral	19–22 years*	25–50 years	51+ years
Vitamin A	5,000 IU †	5,000 IU	5,000 IU
Vitamin D	300 IU	200 IU	200 IU
Vitamin E	15 IU ‡	15 IU	15 IU
Vitamin C	60 mg.	60 mg.	60 mg.
Thiamin	1.5 mg	1.4 mg	1.2 mg.
Riboflavin	1.7 mg	1.6 mg	1.4 mg
Niacin	19 mg.	18 mg.	16 mg.
Vitamin B$_6$	2.2 mg.	2.2 mg.	2.2 mg
Folacin	400 mcg.	400 mcg.	400 mcg.
Vitamin B$_{12}$	3.0 mcg.	3.0 mcg.	3.0 mcg.
Calcium	800 mg.	800 mg.	800 mg.
Phosphorus	800 mg.	800 mg.	800 mg.
Magnesium	350 mg.	350 mg.	350 mg.
Iron	10 mg.	10 mg.	10 mg.
Zinc	15 mg.	15 mg.	15 mg.
Iodine	150 mcg.	150 mcg.	150 mcg.

Sources: *Recommended Dietary Allowance* (National Research Council, 1980); *Handbook of Nonprescription Drugs*, 6th ed. (American Pharmaceutical Association, 1976)
* Vitamins and minerals are described in terms of doses measured in international units (IU), milligrams (mg.) or micrograms (mcg.). A milligram is 1/1000th of a gram; a microgram is 1/1000th of a milligram. The value of an International Unit, on the other hand, may vary from vitamin to vitamin.
† In the future, Vitamin A may be described in units of RE (retinol equivalents). Retinol is the active ingredient in Vitamin A.
‡ In the future, you may find Vitamin E described in units of TE (tocopherol equivalents). Tocopherol is the active ingredient in natural Vitamin E.
§ After menopause, a woman's daily requirement for iron is 10 mg., the same as an adult man's.

Deficiencies and Megadoses That May Affect Fertility

We all need adequate amounts of vitamins and minerals to keep our reproductive system functioning. Too much of one vitamin or too little of another may upset the delicate balance, making a man impotent or a woman unable to conceive.

Vitamin A. This vitamin is essential for the male reproductive system. Without a sufficient supply, a man may not be able to produce sperm. Luckily, vitamin A is stored in body tissues, and a normal, healthy American adult usually has enough in his body to get by for some time even if the vitamin is missing from his diet. That's why vitamin A deficiency is so rare in the United States, usually limited to people who are suffering from some disease or condition that makes it impossible for them to absorb or digest vitamin A. Megadoses of this vitamin may be toxic; they will not cure infertility in an otherwise normal man.

Vitamin D. Vitamin D makes it possible for our bones to absorb and hold calcium; women whose diets do not provide the vitamin D they need may develop osteoporosis that can lead to deformities of the pelvic bones that can make labor and delivery more difficult. Megadoses of this vitamin are potentially poisonous; they may also decrease our desire for sex.

Vitamin E. This vitamin has a totally undeserved reputation as a "fertility tonic," a reputation it gained back in the 1930s when researchers at the University of California discovered that male rats on a vitamin E deficient diet were infertile, and that feeding the rats vitamin E (in the form of vegetable oils) made them fertile again. Megadoses of E, generally considered safe, have no effect whatsoever on the potency or fertility of normal male animals or human beings.

Vitamin B_6. In 1979, *Medical World News* reported that women who had previously been unable to conceive became pregnant after being given 100–800 milligrams of Vitamin B_6 a day (50–400 times the RDA for a normal, healthy woman who is not pregnant). The study was so small, however (14 women), that it is not conclusive. [Note: In 1984, researchers discovered that very large doses of B_6 (2,000–6,000 mg. a day) may cause nerve damage.]

Pantothenic acid. Deficiencies of pantothenic acid have produced many reproductive problems, including infertility, in laboratory animals. The vitamin is found in a wide variety of food, including meat, chicken, whole grains and milk so deficiencies in human beings are almost unknown.

Zinc. Adequate supplies of zinc are essential for sperm production, and it has long been known that men whose diets are moderately to severely deficient in zinc may be unable to produce sperm. They may also suffer from infections, inflammation of the skin, retarded growth and mental slowness. In 1982, researchers at the Wayne State University in Detroit reported that even mild zinc deficiencies too low to be noticed by a physician could affect a man's ability to produce sperm. For six months, volunteers at Wayne State were given a low-zinc diet that forced their bodies to use up the reserves stored in their tissues. As their reserves fell, so did the levels of testosterone in their blood. They lost weight, and their sperm counts fell to the point of infertility. Sperm counts and weight returned to normal when the men went on a high-zinc diet. The Wayne State researchers did not recommend higher doses since zinc interacts with other nutrients and taking more than is necessary may aggravate other marginal deficiencies. In addition, large amounts of zinc (more than 2 grams) cause acute gastrointestinal irritation and vomiting.

Recommendations for Pregnant Women

During pregnancy, a woman's vitamin and mineral requirements increase slightly so that she can provide the nutrients her growing baby needs without depleting her own essential reserves. There is some (slight) controversy as to whether she should get these vitamins and minerals from her food or from a daily supplement, but most people agree on the amounts she will require, basing their recommendations on the 1980 RDAs from the National Research Council's Food and Nutrition Board. The National Research Council updates its recommendations every few years.

Vitamins and Minerals That May Help Prevent Birth Defects

In 1980, British scientists published two important studies suggesting that pregnant women who get a diet containing adequate amounts of vitamins and minerals during the early part of pregnancy

Recommended Daily Dietary Allowances
of Vitamins and Minerals for Pregnant Women

Vitamin/ Mineral	Regular RDA plus:
Vitamin A	+ 1,000 IU
Vitamin D	+ 200 IU
Vitamin E	+ 3 IU
Vitamin C	+ 20 mg.
Thiamin	+ .04 mg.
Riboflavin	+ .03 mg.
Niacin	+ 2 mg.
Vitamin B_6	+ .06 mg.
Folacin	+ 400 mcg.
Vitamin B_{12}	+ 1.0 mcg.
Calcium	+ 400 mg.
Phosphorus	+ 400 mg.
Magnesium	+ 150 mg.
Iron	+ 12–42 mg.*
Zinc	+ 5 mg.
Iodine	+ 25 mcg.

Sources: *Recommended Dietary Allowances* (National Research Council, 1980); *Handbook of Nonprescription Drugs*, 6th ed. (American Pharmaceutical Association, 1976).
* The National Research Council recommends supplemental iron during pregnancy because this amount is rarely supplied by the normal American diet.

may be giving their babies protection against defects of the brain and spinal cord (also known as "neural tube defects").

In the first study, low-income pregnant women who had already given birth to one infant with a neural tube defect (a deformity of the brain or spinal cord) were given vitamin and iron supplements three times a day for at least 28 days before conception occurred and then for at least two months afterward, until the date of the second missed period. (This time period corresponds to the period of time when the fetal brain and nervous system are being formed.) When these women gave birth, the incidence of babies with neural tube defects was lower than expected.

In the second study, the scientists worked with two groups of low-income, high-risk women. The first group was given nutritional counseling (they did not have to follow the advice). The second group got no counseling. When both groups of women gave birth, the researchers found that only women who had not been given nutritional counseling or had not followed their counselor's advice were more likely to give birth to babies with neural tube defects.

It should be noted that in both cases, the supplements and advice aimed to provide only normal amounts of vitamins and minerals, equal to the RDAs. No megadoses were ever prescribed because megadoses of some vitamins and minerals may be hazardous to a developing fetus.

Fluorides for the Fetus?

When we use fluoridated drinking water, some of the fluoride in the water is incorporated into the enamel on our teeth, helping to make them resistant to the acid action that triggers cavities. Some studies have suggested that taking fluoride supplements during pregnancy can enable a mother to give her infant a head start on this kind of cavity-resistance. However, in 1982, the American Dental Association Council on Dental Therapeutics concluded that while there might be a benefit to a child's "baby teeth," the evidence was not strong enough to recommend prenatal fluoride supplements to all prospective mothers. (As has been said so often, there is no evidence at all to suggest that the amounts of fluoride normally found in any municipal water supply will damage either a pregnant woman *or* her fetus.)

Megadoses That May Be Harmful for Your Baby

Megadoses of vitamin A during pregnancy have been linked to deformities of the fetus's ureters (the tube leading from a kidney to the bladder). In 1974, an article in *Obstetrics & Gynecology* described two such cases. In the first, a baby born to a woman who had taken 25,000 IU of vitamin A (five times the RDA for a pregnant woman) every day during the first trimester of her pregnancy and 50,000 IU a day during the second and third trimesters had two ureters (instead of one) attached to one of her kidneys, with the second ureter opening into her vagina. In the second case, a woman who had taken 40,000 IU of vitamin A each day during the sixth to tenth weeks of pregnancy gave birth to an infant with ureters that had no openings at the ends attached to the bladder. In other cases, researchers have suggested that megadoses of vitamin A may be linked to fetal cleft palate, eye damage and webbed fingers or toes.

Large doses of vitamin D may cross the placental barrier, causing hypercalcemia (excess calcium in the blood) in the fetus. In laboratory animals, hypercalcemia may lead to deposits of calcium in soft tissues, including the brain. Calcium deposits in the fetal brain may result in mental retardation. Right now, there is no similar information to show how a pregnant woman's megadoses of vitamin D will affect her fetus.

In one 1972 study, pregnant mice given large doses of vitamin E produced litters with a higher incidence of cleft palate than normal, but in another study, two years later, the offspring of pregnant mice given doses equivalent to 1,000,000 IU for human beings (83,000 times the RDA for pregnant women) showed no ill effects at all.

Women who take large doses of vitamin C while they are pregnant may give birth to babies who temporarily need larger-than-normal doses of vitamin C just to avoid scurvy, the vitamin C deficiency disease. Researchers have suggested that 400–1,000 milligrams a day for a pregnant woman may produce this effect.

Babies born to women who take very large doses of vitamin B_6 while pregnant may also need larger-than-normal amounts to stave off a deficiency.

Deficiencies That May Harm Your Baby

Women who are deficient in vitamin C may pass the deficiency on to the fetus and may give birth to a scorbutic infant (a baby suffering from scurvy).

In experimental animals, maternal deficiency of the B vitamin riboflavin during pregnancy has been linked to cleft palate, heart malformation, lack of growth in the long bones (legs and arms) and eye problems for the newborn.

According to the National Research Council, babies born to women who do not get the recommended 1,200 milligrams of calcium each day while they are pregnant may have bones less dense and strong than they should be. And, in 1983, research from Johns Hopkins University appeared to suggest that a pregnant woman whose diet is deficient in calcium runs a higher-than-normal risk of developing eclampsia late in pregnancy. This condition—high blood pressure, protein in the urine, swelling, convulsions—is responsible for 10% of the maternal deaths and as many as 35% of the stillbirths in this country each year.

Pregnant women who have low blood levels of zinc may be more likely to deliver low-birthweight infants. Zinc, which is found in meat, green leafy vegetables and seafood, interacts with other essential nutrients, including iron. A deficiency (or excess) of one of these nutrients may make it difficult for your body to metabolize another. As a result, some researchers suggest that women who are given iron supplements while they are pregnant may also need zinc supplements. Adequate amounts of zinc may be vital to the proper development of the fetus's immune system. In 1983, researchers at the University of California at Davis reported that mice who do not get enough zinc in the womb seem to have impaired immune function later in life, and their descendants may also have immunological problems.

An Extra Margin of Safety If You Breast-feed

If you plan to breast-feed your infant, you will need extra vitamins and minerals so that you can produce an adequate supply of nutritious milk for your baby without depleting your own body stores of essential nutrients.

Vitamins That May Affect Milk Production

Niacin is a B vitamin found in a wide variety of foods, including meat, fish, chicken, liver, whole-grain cereals and legumes (vegetables such as peas or lima beans whose pods split into two parts with the vegetable attached to one part). A niacin deficiency (which is very rare) may make it difficult to produce milk.

Large doses of vitamin B_6 (also known as pyridoxine) may interfere with milk production. Megadoses of this vitamin are some-

Recommended Daily Dietary Allowances
of Vitamins and Minerals for Women Who Are Breast-Feeding

Vitamin/ Mineral	Regular RDA plus:
Vitamin A	+2,000 IU
Vitamin D	+ 200 IU
Vitamin E	+ 4.5 IU
Vitamin C	+ 40 mg.
Thiamin	+ 0.5 mg.
Riboflavin	+ 0.5 mg.
Niacin	+ 5 mg.
Vitamin B_6	+ 0.5 mg.
Folacin	+ 100 mcg.
Vitamin B_{12}	+ 1.0 mcg.
Calcium	+ 400 mg.
Phosphorus	+ 400 mg.
Magnesium	+ 150 mg.
Iron	+12–42 mg.*
Zinc	+ 10 mg.
Iodine	+ 50 mcg.

Source: *Recommended Dietary Allowances* (National Research Council, 1980).
* Because it is difficult to get this much iron from a normal American diet, the National Research Council recommends iron supplements for women who are breast-feeding.

times used to suppress lactation in women who decide not to breast-feed their infants. The suppressant doses range from 200 to 600 milligrams, more than 100 times the RDA for a normal, healthy adult woman.

Deficiencies That May Make Your Milk Less Nutritious

In most cases, even if you don't get the vitamins and minerals you need each day, your body will go on producing an adequate supply of nutritious milk for your baby, but in the process your own reserves may be depleted. For example, if you don't get the 1,200 milligrams of calcium the National Research Council recommends each day for nursing mothers, your body will put calcium into your milk by taking it out of your bones, a process known as "demineralization." The same thing happens with iron. Your baby is born with a six-month supply of iron stored in her body, so she will have an adequate supply for a while. But your body uses iron to produce milk, so if you do not get the 30–60 milligrams a day the NRC recommends, your own reserves will begin to dwindle.

Deficiencies of vitamin B_1 (thiamin) are rare in healthy people who eat pork, beef, peas, beans, unpolished rice or enriched bread, but if you don't get the 1.5 milligrams you need each day while you are breast-feeding, your infant may develop beriberi, the vitamin B_1 deficiency disease. In a breast-fed infant, any symptoms of a vitamin B_1 deficiency will show up during the second to fourth months. Symptoms of beriberi may include weakness, paralysis and heart failure.

If you are on a strict vegan diet (the form of vegetarianism that excludes all animal products, including milk, cheese and eggs) both you and your infant may be deficient in vitamin B_{12}. Ask your doctor about the value of supplements.

Part VI

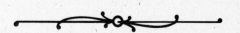

The Environment

19. Where Do You Work?

Until very recently, our concern for how the chemical or physical environment at work might affect our ability to produce healthy babies centered on the danger these things might pose for a pregnant woman and her fetus.

Now, however, we are beginning to learn that these chemicals and conditions may be hazardous for men and women at all stages of their reproductive lives.

Some interfere with the production of sperm. Others may upset a woman's menstrual cycle, making it impossible for her to predict when ovulation will occur. Still others may damage sperm or egg cells so badly that the child they unite to produce is aborted spontaneously—or born with birth defects.

Of course, we still worry about the pregnant woman, because we know that when a working woman is pregnant, her baby shares her exposure to any hazards she faces on the job.

And, there is new concern for the nursing mother, for many industrial chemicals collect in body fat and may pass out of the body in breast milk.

For all these reasons, it is very important that you adhere strictly to any regulations designed to protect women who are or might be pregnant and that you insist that men, too, be protected from the effects of chemical or physical hazards to reproduction.

Chemical and Physical Hazards on the Job

Anesthetic gases. During the 1970s, there were several studies suggesting that the wives of dentists, dental assistants and anesthetists who worked with nitrous oxide ("laughing gas") had a higher-than-normal incidence of spontaneous abortion. In one 1979 study, for example, the rate of miscarriage among wives of dentists working with the anesthetic was 60 percent higher than among wives of

Occupational Hazards to Human Fertility and Reproduction: Who's at Risk?

Hazard	Who May Be at Risk
Anesthetic gases	Dentists, dental assistants, anesthetists, operating room personnel (M)*
Flight	Pilots, cabin attendants (F)
Heat	Bakers, brewers, foundry workers, pottery and ceramics workers, radar and diathermy technicians and operators (M)
Industrial solvents	Artists, auto workers, chemists, art and chemistry teachers, dry cleaners, factory workers, rubber workers, textile workers (M) (F)
Lead	Artists, chemists, art and chemistry teachers, potters and ceramics workers, people who work in plants where paint, roofing material, pipes and lead storage batteries are made, foundry workers or others exposed to smelter emissions (M) (F)
Pesticides	Farm workers, people who work in plants where pesticides are made (M) (F)
Pharmaceuticals	Pharmacists, nurses, people who work in plants where drugs are made (M) (F)
Radiation	People who make nuclear weapons or fuel, people who mine radioactive ore, weld inspectors, radiologists and X-ray technicians (M) (F)

Sources: Chavkin, W., Welch, L., *Occupational Hazards to Reproduction* (The Program in Occupational Health and The Residency Program in Social Medicine, Montefiore Hospital and Medical Center, 1980); Council on Environmental Quality, *Chemical Hazards to Human Reproduction* (National Technical Information Service, January 1981); Dixon, Robert L., Hall, Jerry L., "Reproductive toxicology," *Principles and Methods of Toxicology* (Raven Press, 1982); Thomas, John A., "Reproductive hazards and environmental chemicals: a review," *Toxic Substances Journal*, Vol. 2, No. 4, 1981.
* (M) = male; (F) = female. These evaluations are based on available data and may change as research proceeds.

nondentists. And a 1975 study of male anesthetists in Great Britain showed that they were more likely than men in other professions to father children with minor malformations. Today, none of these studies is regarded as conclusive.

However, more than eight studies since 1970 have shown a significantly higher rate of miscarriage among female doctors, anesthetists, dental assistants and other health care workers who are directly exposed to anesthetic gases at work while they are pregnant. The most extensive of these studies, a 1980 evaluation of questionnaires from more than 30,000 dental assistants, found that the rate of spontaneous abortion was twice as high among the women who had been heavily exposed to nitrous oxide as among the control group of dental assistants who hadn't worked with the nitrous oxide while they were pregnant. There have also been some reports of birth defects (cardiovascular defects, low birthweight) among babies born to women exposed to anesthetic gases during pregnancy.

Cadmium. Cadmium is a toxic metal used in the manufacture of storage batteries. It is also found in smelter emissions. In 1970, a survey of newborns whose mothers had been exposed to cadmium at work while they were pregnant showed an increased incidence of low-birthweight infants. This has not been reported, however, among pregnant women suffering from itai-itai, joint and muscle pains that come with cadmium poisoning. (The name means "ouch, ouch" in Japanese; the condition was first identified in Japan among women who had been eating rice contaminated with cadmium.)

Carbon monoxide. Higher levels of carbon monoxide in the blood of a pregnant woman may interfere with the transport of oxygen to her fetus and may be one explanation for the higher risk of low-birthweight infants among women who smoke or are exposed to the gas at work.

Chloroform. No longer used as an anesthetic, chloroform is still used as an industrial solvent. Pregnant rats exposed to its vapors have been reported to produce low-birthweight infants, and a few have been born with an imperforate anus (an incompletely developed anus with no opening from the body).

Drugs. Many prescription and nonprescription drugs cause reproductive problems, and it is logical to assume that the people who work in the pharmaceutical plants where these drugs are made would suffer from some of these problems. But there is very little research to prove (or disprove) the assumption. In fact, the only conclusive research involves men and women working in plants where oral contraceptives are made. The women working with estrogens often report menstrual irregularities, while the men report decreased libido, and there has been at least one confirmed report of gynecomastia (enlarged breasts) in a male pharmaceutical worker handling estrogens. Hospital personnel are also exposed to drugs, of course. One area of concern may be the nurses, pharmacists and other hospital workers handling cancer drugs, many of which are known to produce chromosomal damage in the patients who take them.

The effects of estrogens on the fetus are well known. There is some possibility that women who work in pharmaceutical plants where oral contraceptives are made may inhale the drugs with which they are working.

Ethylene oxide. Ethylene oxide (EtO) is a sterilizing agent used in hospitals. A 1982 study in the *British Medical Journal* showed that the rate of spontaneous abortion among 1,443 hospital workers exposed to this chemical while they were pregnant was double that among women who, though they also worked in hospitals, were not exposed to EtO.

Flight. A number of scientifically designed studies, including a 1973 study of more than 400 female flight nurses on active duty with the United States Air Force, have validated the informal observation by hundreds of women who work as cabin attendants that frequent flying, particularly on jet aircraft, can cause menstrual irregularities. Sometimes the cycles are longer than normal, sometimes shorter. In both cases, it is more difficult to predict with certainty when ovulation will occur. Once the women stop flying, the situation reverses itself, and the cycles return to normal.

Heat. Under normal circumstances, the temperature in a man's genital area is between 93–95° F. Anything that causes the temperature around the scrotum to rise may affect a man's fertility by slowing or stopping the production of sperm. The men most likely to experience this type of infertility are those who work in foundries or in plants where glass is manufactured or in the engine rooms of ships or in commercial bakeries or on farms. Men who drive trailer trucks over long distances are also at risk since they are exposed to the heat that rises from the engine under or in front of them. Heat-induced infertility is generally only temporary, but in some cases it has lasted for as long as three months after the man was exposed to the very high heat. (See *3. Do You Have an Infectious Disease?*)

People who work with radar or diathermy machines or radio transmitters are also exposed to heat. The microwaves given off by these machines are not ionizing radiation (the kind you get from an X-ray), but they do raise the temperature of any tissues through which they pass.

Lead. Lead is found in many American workplaces. You may be exposed to it if you are an artist or a chemist or teach either of these subjects, or work in a print shop or in a laboratory, or in a plant where pottery or ceramics or paint or storage batteries or pipes or roofing material are made, or if you earn your living as a lead miner or in a factory where you are exposed to smelter emission.

Men who are exposed to lead may be less fertile than others, with lower sperm counts or a higher number of deformed sperm. Sometimes their desire for sex lessens, and, in rare cases, their testicles may atrophy. Their wives may have menstrual irregularities or a higher rate of miscarriage. Women who are exposed to lead at work may also have irregular cycles.

Women who are exposed to lead while they are pregnant have a higher incidence of spontaneous abortion. Their babies, when born alive, are more likely to be low-birthweight or to have birth defects. In 1983, two researchers at Washington University in St. Louis turned up a potential link between a pregnant woman's exposure to lead and her baby's susceptibility to sudden infant death syndrome (SIDS) after birth. Examining the levels of lead in the blood of the umbilical cords of black infants, premature infants and babies born to women who though younger than 19 had more than one child (all three groups are considered at risk for SIDS), the researchers found higher-than-normal levels of lead. The research, though strictly preliminary, may indicate that lead is a factor in SIDS.

Mercury. Like cadmium and lead, this metal may be hazardous for your baby. Methylmercury (an organic mercury compound produced as waste product in pesticide and textile plants) and the vapors of elemental mercury (the kind of mercury used in dental fillings) cross the placenta and may injure the baby's central nervous system, causing brain damage, cerebral palsy, speech problems and tremors. Babies damaged by mercury in their mothers' wombs may be mentally retarded or may develop more slowly physically.

Methyl ethyl ketone. This solvent is widely used in manufacturing chemicals. When pregnant laboratory animals were exposed to its vapors early in pregnancy, their babies were born with a variety of birth defects. Some industrial corporations refuse to permit women of child-bearing age to work in areas where methyl ethyl ketone is used.

Pesticides and herbicides. Laboratory research as well as the experience of people who work on farms or in plants where pesticides and herbicides are manufactured suggests that many of these chemicals can interfere with fertility or cause birth defects when parents are exposed to them before conception occurs.

For example, several studies indicate that carbaryl lowers sperm production in laboratory animals and alters the secretion of hormones that allow the ovaries and testes to grow and function normally.

DBCP has been linked to infertility among the men who have worked in plants where it was made, and a related compound, EDP, may also affect male reproductive function.

DDT lowers sperm production in men and may disrupt the menstrual cycle. In one study of migrant farm laborers, women who complained of menstrual disorders were found to have average blood levels of DDT twice as high as the female farm workers who did not complain of menstrual problems.

Methoxychlor, like chlordecone, seems to interrupt estrogen metabolism in laboratory animals.

2,4,5-T, commonly known as "Agent Orange," and a contaminant called TCDD, a dioxin, are both known to cause birth defects when fed to pregnant rats, hamsters and guinea pigs, but no current research has shown any link to birth defects in other species or among children born to men who were exposed to these chemicals before their children were conceived.

Very small amounts fed to pregnant laboratory rats have killed the fetuses or produced gastrointestinal hemorrhages. Fed to pregnant mice, dioxins have caused fetal cleft palate and kidney malformations. However, tests in nonrodent species, including apes, haven't shown the same sort of damage to the fetus.

Radiation. People who mine radioactive ore, produce nuclear fuel or weapons, check welds or metal equipment (like airplanes) with X-ray scanners, or work as radiologists or X-ray technicians in hospitals or doctors' offices are exposed to higher levels of ionizing radiation than the rest of us are. Altogether, though, they represent a very small population, and there is very little "hard" information on how their radiation exposure affects their fertility or reproductive functions. One 1969 study of female radiologists concluded that they are less fertile than women who work in laboratories or the wives of male radiologists, but the researchers suggest that this may be due to the fact that they are more likely to use birth control. Two studies of male Japanese radiologists, done in 1958 and 1974, also suggest an increased rate of childlessness; 8.4 percent of the men were still childless at the age of 60, a significantly higher rate than found among the rest of the general population in Japan. (For more information on the effects of low-level or small doses of ionizing radiation before conception, see *13. Has Your Doctor Proposed X-Rays?*)

Pregnant women who work near an X-ray machine or in an industry where nuclear materials are used may be exposed to continuous doses of low-level ionizing radiation. The radiation can be extremely hazardous to the fetus, particularly in the very early stages of pregnancy, before you even know you *are* pregnant. Babies who are exposed to radiation while still in the uterus may die in the womb (common only very early in pregnancy), be born with damage to the brain and central nervous system, or be at high risk for childhood cancers.

The question of whether or not the radiation (microwaves)

given off by video display terminals (VDTs) may be harmful to a developing fetus has not yet been conclusively answered. Although there is no proof at all that VDTs are potentially dangerous, there is enough uncertainty among VDT operators to have prompted the National Institute for Occupational Safety and Health to have begun a research project whose results will be announced late in 1987.

Solvents. Benzene, toluene and xylene are solvents (chemicals that dissolve things) found in some art supplies and used in a variety of chemical manufacturing processes. Women exposed to any one of the three may have irregular menstrual cycles; exposure to benzene, a known carcinogen, may lead to chromosomal abnormalities in men or women. Some research on animals showed that the offspring of pregnant rats who were exposed to benzene vapors were likely to grow more slowly than other baby rats and more likely to have malformed bones. Pregnant rats exposed to high concentrations of xylene vapors early in pregnancy also produced infants who grew more slowly than other baby rats, and at least one study has suggested that women who are exposed to toluene vapors while pregnant had an increased risk of producing a low-birthweight baby.

Carbon disulfide is a solvent used to dissolve cellulose, rubber, resins and waxes. It is used in petroleum refining and in the textile industry (to make the semisynthetic fabric rayon). For men, exposure to carbon disulfide may lead to impotence, descreased libido and the production of abnormal sperm. Women exposed to this solvent may have irregular menstrual cycles. Carbon disulfide has also been linked to an increased incidence of miscarriage or premature birth among women who were exposed to its vapors while they were pregnant.

The dry-cleaning solvents, carbon tetrachloride and trichloroethylen (TCE) are known to inhibit sperm production in laboratory rats, and carbon tetrachloride may also inhibit the secretion of a hormone needed for the release of a mature egg from the ovary.

Chloroprene is a solvent used in rubber production. Men who are exposed to it may have lower-than-normal sperm counts; their wives may have an increased risk of miscarriage.

Occupational and Environmental Contaminants in Breast Milk

Many of the industrial and environmental chemicals to which we are exposed are fat-soluble. They are stored in our body fat and rarely excreted except in breast milk.

Perhaps the best-known of the fat-soluble contaminants in breast milk are the polychlorinated biphenyls (PCBs). PCBs are very stable compounds, so stable that they were once used to slow the evaporation of pesticides and prolong their life. Although the Environmental Protection Agency banned the production of PCBs late in the 1970s, fish from the St. Lawrence Seaway and other waters still contaminated by the PCBs dumped there as waste products still contain high levels of these chemicals, and pregnant women who live near these places often have PCBs in their breast milk. How breast milk containing PCBs will affect a nursing infant is a matter of some debate, but some follow-up studies of infants breast-fed by mothers exposed to PCBs have shown neurological and developmental impairment nine years later. The Committee on Environmental Hazards of the American Academy of Pediatrics has advised women who were exposed to these chemicals at work or who have eaten large amounts of fish from PCB-contaminated waters not to breast-feed.

DDT and the related pesticides chlordane, dieldrin, and heptachlor are also stored in body fat and may be excreted in breast milk.

Lead is excreted in breast milk; so is mercury.

Industrial Chemicals in Our Air and Water

Many of the chemicals considered hazardous for pregnant women when we are exposed to them at work end up in our air or water and pose the same risks when we encounter them in everyday life. For example, women who live in neighborhoods near foundries and are exposed to smelter emissions in the air are likely to have the same higher incidence of spontaneous abortion, low-birthweight babies and babies stillborn or born with birth defects as women who work inside the foundries. By the same token, our drinking water may be contaminated with the same pesticides, solvents or other chemicals that are linked to spontaneous abortion, stillbirth or birth defects among women in the workforce. These chemicals make their way into our water as waste products or when they are applied to plants as pesticides and then seep down into the water table. Obviously, all the chemicals in air and water may end up in the food chain. (See *16. Foods That May Contain Hazardous Contaminants.)*

Some Chemicals Known to Be Hazardous for the Fetus That Have Shown Up in the Water Supply in Various Places in the United States

---

Benzene

Chloroform*

DBCP

DDT and related pesticides such as aldrin, dieldrin, heptachlor, chlordane

PCBs

Trichloroethylene (TCE) and related solvents

Radioactive particles†

Vinyl chloride

Sources: Anderson, Duncan, "Poisoned or pure?," *American Health,* July/August 1983, Council on Environmental Quality, *Chemical Hazards to Human Reproduction* (National Technical Information Service, January 1981).

* Formed when chlorine is added to water to minimize bacterial contamination

† From naturally occurring radioactivity in rocks and soil through which the water passes

20. How Safe Is Your Home?

Even if your drinking water is free of industrial chemicals when it gets to your house, it may pick up lead, cadmium and other toxic metals when it travels through lead, galvanized, or polyvinylchloride pipes on the way to your faucet.

Your gas stove and space heater produce carbon monoxide, formaldehyde and other gases as natural waste products when they burn natural gas. If your house is adequately ventilated and your appliances properly adjusted, the levels of these gases (which may be hazardous to the fetus) may be well below the danger level. It is not reassuring to note, however, that our recent attempts to save energy have led some of us to create sealed homes, with the pollutants trapped inside.

Whether or not the amount of radiation released by a properly operated, properly maintained microwave oven is hazardous to the fetus is a matter of some dispute. Several studies have shown that it is not, but many obstetricians and some consumer groups still advise against your using the oven while you are pregnant to avoid even the slightest possibility of fetal damage.

If you are a do-it-yourself person, you may be exposed to solvents and lead compounds in paint, varnish, paint strippers and thinners, and other chemical products used to decorate or repair your home. Some label ingredients to watch out for are benzene, lead compounds, mercury, methyl ethyl ketone, toluene and xylene.

21. Do You Plan to Travel?

Is your destination a problem? Because some live-virus immunizations may be hazardous for a developing fetus, you may have to limit your travel plans, avoiding some countries where immunizations are a necessity.

It's also a good idea to keep in mind the fact that if you are going out of the country you may have a hard time getting the kind of medical attention you will want during pregnancy and delivery. Obviously, this varies with the destination.

How pregnancy may affect your choice of transportation. The days when all visibly pregnant women were banned from passenger planes are long gone, but traveling while you are pregnant may still present some problems on the airlines.

Late in your pregnancy, the airlines become understandably edgy about the possibility of your going into labor in midflight. As a result, some will require you to have your doctor's written permission to travel on board if you are in your eighth month, and a few also require you to have permission to travel during the first week after your baby is born. To avoid unpleasant hassles at the airport, check this out with your travel agent or airline when you make your reservations.

Car travel is convenient, but you are likely to find long trips confining and uncomfortable as your pregnancy progresses.

Ships are roomy and allow you to move about in comfort, but should an emergency occur or should you go into labor late in your pregnancy, you may find yourself far from the kind of medical support you want and need.

Is an airplane cabin safe for pregnant women? In terms of simple convenience, airplanes score low on the list when you are pregnant. For example, you may have to urinate more frequently, but getting to the lavatory and maneuvering around inside—a chore when you're not pregnant—can be even more awkward and uncomfortable now.

On a long flight, you may be sitting in one place for several hours, which may increase your risk of developing thrombophlebitis (blood clots) and edema (swelling). Because of this, some doctors will advise you to avoid all long plane trips while you are pregnant; others may suggest exercising in your seat. You could, for example, flex and unflex your ankles or move around the cabin from time to time during the flight. Like using the lavatory, this can be a problem while you are pregnant. It will be easier, though, to get around a two-aisle jumbo jet than a one-aisle small plane.

The seat belt that keeps you safe in the plane as well as in your own car can be a problem as your girth increases. Most belts are designed to buckle across your stomach, putting pressure on your uterus if the plane lurches or your car stops short, so some experts suggest buckling it around your thighs (under your uterus) rather than around your stomach.

Natural radiation from cosmic rays increases with altitude. People who live in Denver, for example, get about one and a half to two times as much radiation from outer space as do people who live at sea level in New York or Los Angeles. Not unexpectedly, traveling in a jet plane five to eight miles above the earth exposes us to more radiation than most of us get on the ground. For example, the trip from New York to Los Angeles may expose us to about 2.5 millirem of radiation, while the trip from London to Los Angeles may expose us to about 10 millirem. Because this is whole-body exposure, the uterus is exposed to radiation, but the amounts encountered on a single plane trip are approximately several thousand times less than the doses of radiation known to damage or destroy a fertilized egg or fetus. (See *13. Has Your Doctor Proposed X-Rays?*)

Part VII

Tests You Should Know About

22. Tests That Measure Fertility

If you have been trying to become pregnant for a year or more and haven't had any success, your doctor may suggest one of the following tests to find out why.

Tests for Male Fertility

The basic test for male fertility is semen analysis, an examination of the fluid produced by ejaculation. A man's doctor will probably ask him to refrain from intercourse or masturbation for a few days before providing the sample so that sperm counts will be as high as possible. The person who examines the semen sample will consider a number of variables, including:

Texture. A normal semen sample will be sticky, but it should liquify quickly.

Volume. The average amount of semen produced at ejaculation is between one and five milliliters (⅟₃₀–⅙ oz.). More (or less) may indicate infertility.

pH. Normal semen is slightly basic (alkaline), with a pH of 7.2–8. (Acids have a pH lower than 7; bases [alkalis] have a pH higher than 7.)

Sperm count. Most semen samples from fertile men contain 60–120 million sperm in each milliliter of semen. A minimum of 20 million sperm per milliliter is considered essential for conception.

Sperm motility. Sperm must be motile (able to move about actively) in order to make their way through the vaginal mucus and up toward the egg. In a sample of normal semen, at least 60 percent of the sperm will be motile. Sperm motility can be gauged simply by examining a sample of semen under a microscope, or the doctor may use the Huhner test, which involves taking a sample of vaginal mucus immediately after intercourse has occurred to see if the sperm are able to move through the mucus.

Sperm shape. Normal sperm have one head and one tail, and the head is round and smooth. Abnormal sperm may have multiple heads or tails and the head(s) may be oddly shaped. If more than 60 percent of the sperm are oddly shaped, this may be related to infertility and is a signal to proceed with more definitive testing. Sperm with oddly shaped heads may also be linked to birth defects. (See *7. Do you Smoke?; 10. Do You Use Illicit Drugs?; Is the Alcohol You Drink a Hazard?*, p. 91.)

One experimental procedure that may eventually produce a simple, foolproof test for male fertility is the zona-free hamster egg assay. The zona pellucida is a membrane that surrounds mammal eggs and prevents their being fertilized by sperm from another species of animals. Because of the zona pellucida, for example, dogs cannot be impregnated by cats, nor human beings by other animals. For this test, mature eggs are surgically removed from a hamster and then stripped of their zona pellucida. Then they are put into a container with a sample of human semen, and the person running the test watches to see how many sperm from the sample penetrate the hamster eggs after various periods of time ranging from 3 to 24 hours. Researchers at the University of Texas Medical Center in Houston reported in 1983 that men whose sperm were able to penetrate the hamster eggs could reasonably be considered fertile. However, a number of researchers at other laboratories caution that the test (which will not be generally available for some time) is not an absolute measure of human fertility since exceptions occur each time it is run on volunteers who are known to be fertile.

Tests for Female Fertility

In order for a woman to be able to conceive, her body must produce and release a mature egg, the egg must be able to travel from the ovary into the fallopian tube, and the cervical mucus must be "friendly" to the sperm, permitting it to move through the cervix up to where the egg is waiting. There are several tests available to let you and your doctor know whether all these conditions are being met.

Are you ovulating? One way to tell is to keep a chart of your body temperature every day for several months. Your temperature should rise when you ovulate and then stay elevated slightly until right before you begin to menstruate. If this pattern doesn't show up consistently on your temperature chart, you may be ovulating irregularly or not at all.

A second test for ovulation requires you to observe and evaluate your vaginal mucus. Before you ovulate, your vaginal mucus is normally sticky and clear, with a consistency rather like fine honey. After you ovulate, it will thin out and turn milky in color. (At ovulation, some women may observe a small mucus "plug," while others may notice slight bleeding.) NOTE: If you are using a "natural" form of contraception, it is important to remember that while these signs may tell you that you have ovulated, they are not absolute proof against your getting pregnant anyway since some women sometimes produce more than one mature egg during a single monthly cycle.

Can the egg get into the fallopian tube? The Rubin test is one way to find out. For this procedure, your doctor will introduce some carbon dioxide (CO_2) into your uterus. If your fallopian tubes are clear, not blocked by scars or other defects, the gas will rise through them into your abdominal cavity. Your doctor can hear the gas escaping when she presses a stethoscope against your abdomen; you can tell what's happening when you feel a sudden pain in your shoulder that lets you know that the gas has moved into the abdominal cavity and is pressing against your diaphragm.

The Rubin test is very helpful, but it will not let your doctor know if there is a partial blockage in one or both tubes or if one tube is entirely blocked. A hysterosalpingogram is required to give her this kind of specific information. For this X-ray procedure, a dye is injected into the uterus and allowed to flow upward through the fallopian tubes. If the tubes are clear, the dye will show that clearly.

A third, more complicated procedure, is laparoscopy. Laparoscopy is surgery, performed under a general anesthetic. Your doctor makes a tiny incision in your abdomen and inserts a small viewing device. Then dye is inserted into your uterus through your vagina, and your doctor watches to see if the dye eventually spills out of the top of the fallopian tubes into the abdominal cavity, indicating that the tubes are free of obstructions.

Is your cervical mucus "friendly" to your partner's sperm? If you take a sample of cervical mucus from a fertile woman who is ovulating and spread it on a glass slide, when you look at it under a microscope you will see that it has dried in a distinctive pattern that looks something like a fern leaf, with lots of tiny little channels. The ferning pattern (which indicates high estrogen) is the basis for the postcoital test. This test is done when you are ovulating. A sample of vaginal mucus is taken as soon after intercourse as possible. If the fern pattern appears when the mucus is observed under a microscope, and if there are many live sperm swimming around on the slide, the test shows that mucus and sperm are compatible. (It is also a guide to the quality and quantity of mobile sperm in the ejaculate.)

23. Genetic Screening

If you or your partner or someone in either of your families has an inherited birth defect or disorder, a genetic counselor can help you figure out the chances of your passing the problem on to any children you may have.

Ethnic Origins and Inherited Genetic Disorders

If You Are:	There Is an Increased Risk That You May Be Carrying the Gene For*
Black	*Lactase deficiency:* a lack of the enzyme that makes it possible to digest lactose, the sugar in milk and milk products.
	Sickle cell anemia: a disorder of the red blood cells in which the cells are oddly shaped ("sickled") and have a hard time getting through small blood vessels. As a result, they may pile up (clump) at the entrance to blood vessels. Because the sickled cells are fragile, they may also break as they travel around the body.
	Cooley's anemia: a blood disorder, also known as beta-thalassemia, which may cause enlargement of the liver and spleen, jaundice, stones in the gall bladder, thickening of the skull bones that produces a characteristically "thickened" face and death before the age of 30.
Chinese	*Lactase deficiency:* see above, under *Black*.
	alpha-Thalassemia: an anemia resulting from an inability to synthesize hemoglobin properly; this form of thalassemia may kill the fetus before it is born or may be fatal for the newborn baby.

Ethnic Origins and Inherited Genetic Disorders (*cont.*)

If You Are:	*There Is an Increased Risk That You May Be Carrying the Gene For**
English	*Neural tube defects:* defects of the spinal column. One well-known neural tube defect is spina bifida, a condition in which the spinal column remains open instead of closing tight.
Greek	*Cooley's anemia:* see above, under *Black.*
	Glycogen storage disease, Type III: an enzyme deficiency that interferes with the body's ability to break down glycogen, the form in which sugar is stored in the liver until needed for energy. As a result, abnormal amounts of gylcogen build up in the liver as well as in the muscle and heart tissues.
Irish	*Neural tube defects:* see above, under *English.*
Italian	*Cooley's anemia:* see above, under *Black.*
	Glycogen storage disease, Type III: see above, under *Greek.*
Japanese	*Dyschromatosis:* unusual pigmentation of the skin that may occur in small patches or all over the body.
	Oguchi's disease: night blindness.
Jewish—Eastern European	*Bloom's syndrome:* reddened marks on face, hands and arms caused by dilated blood vessels; dwarfism.
	Gaucher's disease: an inability to metabolize fat that results in enlargement of the liver and spleen, pigmentation of the skin and, often, death within a year of birth.
	Meckel's syndrome: a group of birth defects, including cleft palate, sloping forehead, deformed kidneys and eye defects; usually proves fatal soon after birth.

Ethnic Origins and Inherited Genetic Disorders (*cont.*)

If You Are:	There Is an Increased Risk That You May Be Carrying the Gene For*
	Niemann-Pick disease: an enzyme deficiency that makes it impossible to metabolize fat properly and causes enlarged liver and spleen and mental retardation.
	Tay-Sachs disease: one of a group of inherited conditions that cause spastic paralysis, blindness, convulsions, mental deterioration and death, usually very early in life.
	Ziehan-Oppenheim disease: a disorder characterized by muscle spasms that progressively distort the shape of the spine and hips.
Jewish—Sephardic (Mediterranean)	*Cooley's anemia:* see above, under *Black.*
	Glycogen storage disease, Type III: see above, under *Greek.*
Korean	*Dyschromatosis:* see above, under *Japanese.*
	Oguchi's disease: see above, under *Japanese.*
South African—white	*Variegate porphyria:* skin sensitivity to light.

Sources: McCormack, Michael K., "Medical genetics and family practice," *American Family Physician,* September 1979; *The Merck Manual,* 14th ed. (Merck, Sharp & Dohme, 1982); *Stedman's Medical Dictionary,* 24th ed. (Williams & Wilkins, 1982).

24. Carrier Tests

In some cases, your genetic counselor may recommend a blood test to find out whether you are carrying a genetic disorder even if you show no signs of it yourself. These tests—known as carrier tests—may be suggested routinely if you are a member of a group known to be at high risk for a particular condition. Black people may be tested for sickle cell anemia. Jews of Eastern European origin may be tested for Tay-Sachs disease, Gaucher's disease, and Niemann-Pick disease. Greeks and others from the Mediterranean area may be tested for Cooley's anemia. In other cases, because the actual test is more complicated (for the technician, not for you), testing will be suggested only if you are known to be at risk, that is, if someone in your family has had the disorder or if you have shown signs of it. Hemophilia and other clotting disorders fall into this category. So do the chromosomal abnormalities that may cause multiple miscarriage or a relatively rare kind of Down's syndrome.

Because research into genetic disorders is proceeding at a rate that produces enormous jumps in knowledge, it is always best to check with your own physician or genetic counselor. New information or tests pertinent to your particular needs may show up at any moment.

25. Testing for Rubella Antibodies

In children, rubella (which is also known as "German measles") is a mild infection that leaves no lasting effects. For pregnant women, however, it can be a disaster. The rubella virus crosses the placenta. It may infect the fetus and, if it does, it can cause a variety of serious birth defects including loss of hearing, cataracts and other eye damage, damage to the heart and skeletal muscles and mental retardation. Rubella is most dangerous early in pregnancy. Sixty percent of the babies whose mothers catch rubella during the first eight weeks of pregnancy will be infected, and 80 percent of them will be born with birth defects that show up right away or as the babies grow older. Later in pregnancy, rubella is less threatening to the developing fetus. For example, if a pregnant woman catches it after the twentieth week of pregnancy, even if her baby is infected, no ill effects are likely.

If you don't know for sure whether or not you have already had rubella, your doctor can find out with a simple blood test that looks for antibodies in your blood. (Antibodies show that you once had the infection and that your body mobilized to fight it. They are your protection against reinfection.) If you don't have any antibodies, you can be immuzined against rubella. Since the vaccine that is used to immunize you will contain live virus, many doctors stress caution, suggesting that you should not take the vaccine while you are pregnant, and that you should wait two to three months after being vaccinated before becoming pregnant. Because there is some question as to exactly how long the immunity conferred from the vaccination will last, ask your doctor if you need to be retested and reimmunized the next time you decide to become pregnant. From a public health standpoint, protection against rubella is very important to get; the disease is much more common than many other causes of birth defects, and thus your chances of being exposed to it are greater.

26. Testing for Toxic Metals

If you or your partner have been exposed to high levels of arsenic, cadmium, lead, mercury or any other metal that can affect your ability to conceive or carry a healthy baby, your doctor may suggest tests that determine just how much of these toxic metals you have stored in your body. The simplest screening tests are hair analysis and fingernail analysis. Both your hair and your nails contain all the metals found in your body, and if the amounts are suspiciously high, your doctor may suggest further tissue analyses to get more precise measurements. However, because there is much debate as to the reliability of these tests, they are normally suggested only for people who are involved in occupations or recreational activities (hobbies) that expose them to high levels of toxic metals.

27. Pregnancy Detection Tests

When you are pregnant, the chorion (a membrane around the fetus that eventually becomes part of the placenta) begins to produce human chorionic gonadotrophin (HCG), a hormone that prevents menstruation and allows the pregnancy to continue. All modern pregnancy tests, from the simplest to the most sophisticated, are designed to detect the presence (or absence) of HCG in your body.

The Ascheim-Zondek ("A-Z") test, created by two German researchers in the 1920s, requires the person running the test to inject a sample of a potentially pregnant woman's urine into a laboratory rabbit, which is then sacrificed. If the woman is pregnant, the HCG in her urine will set off changes in the rabbit's ovaries that are clearly visible when the animal is dissected. Because rabbits are expensive, rats are often substituted. When they are, the test is known as the Friedman test.

For the most part, these pregnancy detection tests involving animals have been replaced by quicker, cheaper, immunological tests that measure the reaction between HCG in your blood or urine and HCG antibodies on latex particles or animal red blood cells.

Pregnancy test kits for home use come equipped with a small sample of red blood cells (usually from a sheep) coated with HCG antibodies, to which you add a small amount of your own urine. If there is a high enough concentration of HCG in your urine, it will agglutinate (clump) the HCG antibodies, forming the "doughnut" or ring that serves to indicate that you are pregnant.

These home test kits are not infallible. For one thing, they are not sensitive enough to catch very small amounts of HCG, so if you use them too early in your pregnancy, they may produce a false-negative result, suggesting that you aren't pregnant when you really are. If the container for the test is not perfectly clean, or if you move the test while it is working, or if you have a vaginal or urinary infection, or if you are using some psychiatric drugs (e.g., chlordi-azepoxide [Librium], chlorpromazine [Thorazine]), oral contraceptives or methadone, or if you have an ectopic pregnancy or one that is about to miscarry, you may also get a false-negative result. On the other hand, if you are near menopause, or have a uterine cancer, or have recently been pregnant, you may get a false-positive result because all these conditions alter the balance of hormones in your body. Waiting too long to read the test can also give you a false-positive result.

The most reliable pregnancy detection test is the radioassay immunological test, in which the HCG antibodies are mixed with HCG that has been tagged with radioactive isotopes. This works very quickly and it can detect a pregnancy within a few days of conception. It is most accurate if given at the time of your first missed period.

28. Prenatal Medical Tests

Blood tests. Blood tests are a routine part of a pregnant woman's prenatal medical regime. They are used to screen for warning signals or to diagnose conditions that may be hazardous for the fetus.

AFP. Alpha fetoprotein (AFP) is a protein produced by the fetus. AFP never shows up in a healthy adult's blood except during pregnancy or as a warning signal for certain kinds of cancer. While you are pregnant, it is normal to have small amounts of this protein in your blood. Higher levels may indicate more than one fetus in the womb or a low-birthweight baby or a baby with a neural tube defect or one that has died in the uterus. AFP is also found in amniotic fluid, and, until 1983, amniocentesis was the only way to measure its presence. The Food and Drug Administration has now approved a simple blood test for AFP. It is important to remember that the AFP test is only an indicator. It is not a conclusive proof of damage to the fetus, because high levels of AFP can occur in benign conditions (when you are carrying twins, for example) as well as in dangerous ones. If you have high levels of AFP in your blood, your doctor will *always* call for more sophisticated tests (sonography, amniocentesis) to find out why.

Estriol. Estriol is a metabolite (by-product) of estrogen. The placenta produces estriol, and when you are pregnant the level of estriol in your blood will rise steadily until the last three months of pregnancy, when it should level out and remain steady until your baby is born. As long as this pattern is present, your doctor will assume that your baby is growing safe and well. If your estriol levels begin to fall, though, your doctor will immediately try to find out why. (If you are a diabetic, falling estriol levels may be a signal to deliver the baby as quickly as possible.)

Infectious diseases. In many states, the law requires your doctor to test your blood for syphilis antibodies on your first prenatal visit. Blood tests can also show the presence of rubella antibodies, letting your doctor know that you are already immune to rubella.

Blood pressure readings. Your doctor will keep a close check on your blood pressure while you are pregnant because rising pressure may warn of pre-eclampsia. (Higher-than-normal levels of uric acid in your blood may be another warning of pre-eclampsia.)

Urinalysis. Urinalysis offers your doctor a second means of monitoring estriol levels in your body. Bacterial counts can show if you are developing a urinary infection, and diabetics can use urine tests to monitor their own condition (the level at which the kidneys begin to "spill" sugar into the urine is lower when you are pregnant). Finally, urinalysis offers your doctor a chance to monitor levels of uric acid that may serve as another indicator of possible pre-eclampsia.

Tissue cultures for sexually transmitted diseases. Secretions or tissues from the vaginal or genital area can be cultured to test for the sexually transmitted diseases chlamydia, gonorrhea and herpes.

Sonography. Sonography is the use of sound waves to create a picture. To show the fetus inside your womb, a technician presses a transducer (which looks something like a small, square box) against your abdomen. The transducer sends short bursts of sound waves through the abdominal wall into your womb. Inside the amniotic sac, the sound waves bounce around through the amniotic fluid. Every time they hit the fetus's body, an electrical impulse is transmitted to the sonograph, the televisionlike machine on which the sonogram (picture) appears. The sonogram shows the fetus clearly, and most prospective parents find this first view of their baby an overwhelming emotional experience. For the doctor, it is extremely informative. The sonogram lets him know right away if there is more than one baby in the womb. It outlines any defects in the fetal skeleton and shows cysts and tumors, as well as any masses in the baby's body that may indicate a malformation or malfunction of the intestinal or urinary tract. A sonogram shows the fetal heart beat, and as your pregnancy goes on, repeated sonograms allow your doctor to monitor your baby's growth and, eventually, her readiness to be born. (Sonograms also show the position and condition of the placenta.)

The most remarkable thing about sonography is that it does all this without the ionizing radiation known to damage body cells and chromosomes. Most studies have shown no problems for the developing fetus. However, because the technique is so new, there simply is no conclusive evidence as to whether or not it really is safe for the baby.

As a result, there is growing sentiment that sonography should not be used routinely or casually (for example, to provide a picture for the family scrapbook). In 1984, a Consensus Panel at the National Institutes of Health set up some tentative guidelines for the conservative use of sonography during pregnancy.

These are some of the conditions the panel felt might necessitate the use of sonography:

- when the doctor suspects a woman may be carrying more than one baby
- when a woman becomes pregnant with an IUD in place (sonography can help the doctor pinpoint the device so that it can be removed)
- when the doctor suspects an ectopic pregnancy
- when the doctor suspects that the fetus has died or may be malformed
- when there is a possibility that the placenta may be damaged or abnormal
- when there is an unusual pelvic mass
- when a pregnant woman has vaginal bleeding for which there is no apparent cause
- to evalute the health of the fetus when a woman does not get prenatal care until late in her pregnancy
- when the baby may be in a breech position and this cannot be determined by manual examination
- when a doctor may need to perform a cesarean delivery or induce labor and must have a good idea of the fetus's age and development

Amniocentesis. Inside the uterus, the fetus floats in a fluid-filled sac that protects it against shocks from outside its mother's body.

The sac is formed by a membrane called the amnion, and the fluid is called amniotic fluid.

Amniotic fluid is a wonderful source of information about your growing baby because it contains cells from the fetus's body. It may also contain traces of enzymes or other substances that alert your doctor to the possibility that your baby may have a congenital or inherited disorder.

By the sixteenth week of pregnancy, there is sufficient fluid in the amniotic sac for your doctor to be able to pass a long hollow needle through your abdominal wall into the uterus and withdraw a sample. The doctor will be careful to avoid hitting the fetus, which has been located via sonography (see p. 144). This drawing of a sample of amniotic fluid is called amniocentesis (centesis means "puncture"). It poses some risks for the fetus; in about 1 in every 300 cases, a miscarriage will follow. In addition, since it may take as long as four weeks to perform some of the tests on cells from the amniotic fluid, this procedure can be hard to deal with psychologically. Amniocentesis is not done routinely in every pregnancy, nor should it be. Rather, it is reserved for pregnancies in which it is important to learn as much about the baby as possible. Some examples are:

- when the pregnant woman is older than 30
- when she has already given birth to an infant with a neural tube defect such as spina bifida or some other congenital defect such as renal agenesis (the absence of one or both kidneys)
- when she has already given birth to an infant with a form of mental retardation linked to a chromosomal abnormality
- when she is a diabetic; often, infants born to diabetic women must be delivered before they have reached full term, and analysis of amniotic fluid allows the physician to find out whether the baby's lungs are mature enough to make safe delivery possible
- when either mother or father is a known carrier of an inherited disorder that can be diagnosed through amniocentesis; in some cases, the physician may use amniocentesis even though the test cannot diagnose the inherited condition in the child (for example, if the mother is known to carry an X

chromosome-linked condition such as one form of muscular dystrophy, the doctor may use amniocentesis to determine the sex of the child; males are much more likely than females to inherit an X-linked defect.)

- when either mother or father has a genetic disorder, even in a mild form, that might show up in a more severe form in their child

Chorion biopsy. Inserting a catheter through your cervix, your doctor may soon be able to collect a sample of tissue from the chorion, a membrane surrounding the amniotic sac that eventually becomes part of the placenta. Examining fetal cells from the chorion makes it possible to pinpoint possible congenital malformations and genetic defects. Unlike amniocentesis, this test can be performed very early in pregnancy (as early as the seventh week), and the results may be made available overnight. First used in 1983 at Michael Reese Hospital in Chicago, chorion biopsy may not yet be widely available, and information as to its safety is very preliminary. Some concern has been raised by a 1984 study which suggested that the rate of miscarriage associated with chorion biopsy may be as high as 8–9 percent.

Fetoscopy. For this procedure, a fiberoptic endoscope (a thin, flexible viewing tube) called a fetoscope is inserted through your abdominal wall directly into the uterus. Fetoscopy gives the surgeon an unprecedented chance to look directly at the fetus inside the womb, although the viewing field is very small (it may be blocked entirely by the hand of an 18-week fetus) and can be obscured by blood or meconium (fetal wastes) in the amniotic fluid. During fetoscopy, the doctor may take a sample of fetal blood or skin, allowing her to diagnose congenital blood disorders like thalassemia or sickle cell anemia or congenital dermatological problems like icthyosis congenita (dry skin with fishlike scales). Fetoscopy is a risky procedure, used in cases in which there is no other way to confirm a suspected congenital abnormality.

Finding Birth Defects Before the Baby Is Born

Condition	MATERNAL BLOOD TEST OR URINALYSIS	SONOGRAPHY	AMNIOCENTESIS	FETOSCOPY
Screening or Diagnostic Tests That Have Been Used to Detect This Condition*				
Skull and brain				
Anencephaly (missing brain or skull)	X	X	X	X
Open skull and spinal cord		X	X	X
Dandy-Walker syndrome (fluid in brain)		X		
Enlarged, fluid-filled skull		X		
Encephalocele (gap in the skull)		X	X	
Abnormally small brain (microcephaly)		X		
Spinal cord				
Spina bifida (spinal column that has not closed properly)	X	X	X	X
Heart				
Irregular heartbeat		X		
Enlarged aorta		X		
Enlarged ventricle (chamber of the heart)		X		
Acardia (missing heart)		X		
Skeleton				
Dwarfism		X		
Amelia (missing limbs)		X		
Phocomelia (missing long bones; hands and feet attached directly to shoulders or hips)		X		

Finding Birth Defects Before the Baby Is Born (*cont.*)

Condition	Screening or Diagnostic Tests That Have Been Used to Detect This Condition*			
	MATERNAL BLOOD TEST OR URINALYSIS	SONOGRAPHY	AMNIOCENTESIS	FETOSCOPY
Gastrointestinal tract				
Absence of normal opening from the esophagus			X	
Absence of normal opening from the duodenum		X	X	
Absence of normal opening from the anus		X	X	
Liver growing outside the fetal body		X		
Internal organs, outside the fetal body, in a sack formed by the base of the umbilical cord	X	X	X	
Obstruction in the gastrointestinal tract	X	X		
Urinary tract				
Missing kidneys		X		
Enlarged (polycystic) kidneys		X		
Kidney disease			X	
Metabolic disorders				
Inability to metabolize proteins			X	
Inability to metabolize carbohydrates (galactosemia, Pompe's disease)			X	
Inability to metabolize starches (Hunter syndrome, Hurler syndrome)			X	
Inability to metabolize fats (Fabry's disease, Farber disease, Gaucher's disease, Niemann-Pick disease, Tay-Sachs disease)			X	
Lack of enzyme needed to metabolize phosphates		X	X	
Pituitary hormone deficiency			X	

Finding Birth Defects Before the Baby Is Born (*cont.*)

Condition	MATERNAL BLOOD TEST OR URINALYSIS	SONOGRAPHY	AMNIOCENTESIS	FETOSCOPY
Blood disorders				
Erythroblastosis fetalis (anemia of newborn in which red blood cells are destroyed)		X	X	
Hemophilia				X
Sickle cell anemia			X	X
alpha-Thalassemia		X	X	X
Tumors and cysts				
All		X		
Chromosomal abnormalities				
Down's syndrome caused by an additional chromosome			X	
Extra set of chromosomes (triploidy)			X	
One extra chromosome			X	
Missing chromosomes			X	
Skin disorders				
Icthyosis (dry, scaly skin)				X
Extreme sensitivity to ultraviolet light			X	
General conditions of fetus				
More than one fetus	X	X		
Ectopic pregnancy	X	X		
Low birthweight or retarded growth		X	X	

Screening or Diagnostic Tests That Have Been Used to Detect This Condition

Finding Birth Defects Before the Baby Is Born (*cont.*)

Condition	Screening or Diagnostic Tests That Have Been Used to Detect This Condition*			
	MATERNAL BLOOD TEST OR URINALYSIS	SONOGRAPHY	AMNIOCENTESIS	FETOSCOPY
General conditions of fetus (cont.)				
Misplaced or deformed placenta		X		
Muscular dystrophy (Duchenne's)			X	
Death of the fetus	X	X	X	

Sources: *The Merck Manual,* 14th ed. (Merck, Sharpe & Dohme, 1982); Pinckney, Cathey; Pinckney, Edward, *The Patient's Guide to Medical Tests* (Facts on File, 1982); *Stedman's Medical Dictionary,* 24th ed. (Williams & Wilkins, 1982); Stephenson, Sharon R.; Weaver, David R., "Prenatal diagnosis—a compilation of diagnosed conditions," *American Jouranl of Obstetrics and Gynecology,* October 1, 1981.

* In some cases, tests may not be in general use or may be restricted to high-risk individuals.

29. Tests That Start after Labor Begins

Fetal monitoring. When labor starts, your doctor may begin to record your baby's heartbeat and to measure the strength of your contractions. This procedure, which is called fetal monitoring, is designed to give early warning of any problems your baby may be encountering and predict the delivery of the baby. At first, your doctor will check the baby's heartbeat every 15 or 30 minutes. As labor progresses, the check will be made every 15 minutes, and just before delivery, the heartbeat will be monitored after every contraction. It is possible to do this manually, by applying a stethescope to your abdomen, but many hospitals now prefer to use electronic instruments, which are more sensitive and, many think, more reliable. An external electronic monitor consists of two belts wrapped around your abdomen. Each belt contains a device that sends impulses to a recording machine. One device records the baby's heartbeat; the other, the strength of your contractions. After your membranes rupture and your cervix begins to dilate, an internal electronic monitor may be inserted. This monitor consists of an electrode attached to the baby's scalp (to record the heartbeat) and a plastic tube filled with fluid (to give an indication of how strong your contractions are).

People who favor electronic monitoring point out that half of all the babies who develop problems or die during delivery give no hint of trouble beforehand. They also point out that an electronic monitor works all the time. It won't miss something because it has to leave the room for a minute. On the other hand, people who oppose electronic monitoring stress the fact that doctors may misinterpret the data it provides. Not all babies with an irregular heartbeat are actually in danger, and doctors who hasten delivery to save a "threatened" baby may actually be endangering a healthy one. To avoid this possibility, doctors now follow up suspicious heartbeats with a test of a sample of blood from the baby's scalp. If the blood is oxygen-deficient, the baby may be in trouble.

30. Tests for the Newborn

The Apgar Score. Within a minute after birth, your doctor will add up your baby's first Apgar Score. This measures her respiratory function by observing five specific variables: skin tone (color), heartbeat, breathing, muscle tone and reflexes (how your baby reacts when a catheter is inserted into her nose). If your baby's body is pink all over, if she has a heartbeat above 100, is breathing well and crying, moves about actively and sneezes or coughs when the catheter is inserted, she gets two points for each variable—a total score of 10. If her body is pink but her hands and feet are blue, her heartbeat is under 100, she is breathing slowly or irregularly, just bends her hands and feet and only grimaces at the catheter, she gets one point for each sign. No points at all are given for a blue, pale body, a lack of heartbeat or breathing, limp hands, feet, arms and legs, and no response to the catheter. The test will be repeated five minutes after birth. Few infants get a 10; a score below 4 on the second test may indicated lasting damage or early death. But some infants with a low score do live and flourish.

Genetic screening for the newborn baby. If either you or your partner is a carrier or member of a group known to be at high risk for sickle cell anemia, thalassemia, hemophilia or galactosemia, your baby will also be considered high-risk. In some states, testing high-risk newborns for sickle cell anemia and galactosemia is mandatory. And, even where it is not required by law, some hospitals now test all high-risk newborns for these two inherited disorders, as well as for thalassemia and hemophilia. In all cases, only simple blood tests are required. In virtually all modern hospitals, every newborn will be given the simple blood or urine test for PKU (phenylketonuria).

Testing for infectious diseases. This is also a routine part of neonatal care in many states, because infants born with congenital rubella may not show any signs of infection at birth. The same is true of babies with toxoplasmosis; as many as 70 percent of the babies born with a congenital form of this parasitical infection won't show any signs of it at birth. Found early, toxoplasmosis can be treated through the first year of the baby's life to minimize its long-term effects.

If you have chlamydia, gonorrhea or an active case of genital herpes, your baby may pick up the infection when she travels down the vaginal tract. To avoid this, your doctor may take samples of your vaginal tissues late in pregnancy to see if you have one of these infections and should deliver by cesarean. These tests take anywhere from several hours to several days to complete, but in the near future, tests that can be read in a matter of minutes may be available, allowing your obstetrician to decide at the very last minute whether it is safe to allow a vaginal delivery or whether a cesarean delivery is required.

31. Tests for Breast-feeding Mothers

Measuring the prolactin levels in your blood. Prolactin is a pituitary hormone that stimulates milk production. If you are having difficulty producing milk, there is a simple blood test that will let your doctor know if you are deficient in prolactin. Tranquilizers, antidepressants and some hypertension medication can lower your body levels of this hormone.

Testing for industrial or environmental contaminants. If you have been exposed to PCBs, DDT and other fat-soluble pesticides or certain toxic metals present in the workplace (and sometimes in the environment), the presence of these contaminants can be detected in your breast milk. If they are there, your doctor may advise you not to nurse your infant.

Glossary

Abortion. Birth or termination of a pregnancy before the baby is able to live on its own outside its mother's womb. Usually this means before the twentieth week of pregnancy or when the baby weighs less than 500 grams (about 17 oz.). An *induced abortion* is one brought on by drugs or a medical procedure designed to end the pregnancy; a *spontaneous abortion* (sometimes called a *miscarriage*) is one that occurs naturally.

Amenorrhea. The absence of menstruation. *Primary amenorrhea* means that menstrual periods have never occurred; *secondary amenorrhea* means that menstruation has stopped due to drugs, stress or some other influence.

Aphrodisiac. Something that increases sexual desire.

Birth defect. A malformation or imperfection present at birth.

Chromosome. A body in the nucleus of a living cell on which genes are located. Normal human beings have 46 chromosomes in each cell.

Conception. The fertilization of an egg by a sperm.

Congenital birth defect. A defect present at birth. Congenital birth defects may be hereditary (passed on through the genes), or they may occur during pregnancy due to drugs or some other teratogen, or they may occur during deliver.

Delivery. The movement of the baby from the vaginal canal into the world.

Edema. The accumulation of watery fluid in cells under the skin. Edema causes swelling. In pregnancy, edema in the legs and ankles is common.

Ejaculation. The release of seminal fluid during orgasm.

Embryo. An individual during its earliest stages of life, from conception until about the end of the second month of pregnancy.

Fertility. The ability to produce children. In men, this means the ability to provide viable sperm that can fertilize an egg. In women, it means the ability to provide a mature egg and make it available to the sperm.

Fertilization. The penetration of the egg by the sperm and the combining of these two cells so as to produce a new individual.

Fetus. An individual from the third month of pregnancy until birth.

Gene. A structure on a chromosome that carries hereditary characteristics such as eye and hair color, body size and build, and genetic disorders such as hemophilia, thalassemia and Tay-Sachs disease.

Genetic disorder. A hereditary defect.

Genetic mutation. A permanent alteration in the genetic material that is passed on to new cells whenever the cell in which the damaged gene is located reproduces itself.

Hereditary birth defect. Something that can be passed on from parent to child through the genes.

High-risk. A phrase used to describe individuals who are more likely than most to be born with or develop certain genetic or other problems. Black children, for example, are considered high-risk when it comes to sickle cell anemia, while low-birthweight infants are high-risk when it comes to respiratory problems.

Implantation. The attachment of a fertilized egg to the lining of the uterus. If the egg attaches itself to other tissue, the resulting pregnancy is called *ectopic* (*ec* = "outside"; *topic* = "the place").

Impotence. The inability to attain an erection. Impotent men are not necessarily infertile.

Infertility. The inability to produce a baby. A man may be infertile because his sperm count is low or the sperm he produces are not active and healthy. A woman may be infertile because she does not ovulate or because an obstruction in her fallopian tube prevents the egg and sperm from meeting.

Labor. The process by which the baby comes out of the uterus and down the vaginal canal and is born.

Lactation. The production of milk for a nursing infant.

Libido. The desire for sex.

Low-birthweight. Generally used to describe a baby who weighs less than five pounds at birth. Low-birthweight babies are more likely than others to have trouble breathing and to experience other difficulties because their bodies are not fully developed.

Menstruation. The regular, periodic shedding of the lining of the uterus accompanied by a flow of bloody fluid. Normally, the bleeding (the *menses*) comes about two weeks after ovulation, but some women may bleed without having ovulated. The bleeding experienced by women using oral contraceptives is not menstruation; women on The Pill neither ovulate nor menstruate.

Miscarriage. A spontaneous abortion.

Motile. Able to move about actively. Men whose sperm are not motile are often infertile.

Mutagen. Anything that alters genetic material inside a living cell.

Ovulation. The release of a mature egg from the ovary.

Placenta. The tissue through which a pregnant woman supplies oxygen and nutrients to her fetus and the fetus expels some wastes (notably carbon dioxide). Some drugs and other harmful substances cross the placenta. After delivery, the placenta, now known as the *afterbirth,* is expelled from the mother's body.

Pregnancy. The time from the moment after conception until the child is born.

Prenatal. Referring to the period before birth, as in *prenatal care.*

Premature. A premature baby is one born before 37 weeks, the length of a normal pregnancy.

Potency. The ability to attain an erection. Potency and fertility are different things; a potent man may or may not be fertile, and vice versa.

Semen. The fluid containing the semen; the *ejaculate.*

Sterility. An inability to have children. Sterility connotes a more permanent conditon than infertility.

Teratogen. Anything that causes abnormal development of a fetus. The word comes from the Greek word for monster (*teras*) and generally refers to drugs or chemicals that cross the placenta.

Where to Go for More Information

This is a partial listing of the organizations and agencies that provide information and sometimes counseling on issues related to conception, pregnancy and childbirth. Because these groups sometimes hold opposing views, the information you get may be contradictory. When that happens, your own doctor (who is familiar with your medical history and your attitudes toward child-bearing) is your best source of unbiased evaluation. It goes without saying, of course, that you should *never* act on medical advice from an outside organization without seeking your doctor's advice.

Abortion (Policy Information)

National Organization for Women
425 Thirteenth Street NW
Washington, D.C. 20004
(202) 347-2279

National Right to Life
Suite 402
419 Seventh Street NW
Washington, D.C. 20004
(202) 638-4650

Planned Parenthood Federation of
  America
2010 Massachusetts Avenue NW
Washington, D.C. 20036
(202) 785-3351

Birthing Centers

The National Association of
  Childbirth Centers
Box 1
Route 1
Perkiomenville, Pa. 18074
(215) 234-8068

Chemicals

Chemical Manufacturers
  Association
2501 M Street NW
Washington, D.C. 20037
(202) 887-1100

Consumer Health Issues

The American Council on Science
and Health
47 Maple Street
Summit, N.J. 07901
(201) 277-0024
1995 Broadway
New York, N.Y. 10023
(212) 362-7044

The Center for Science in the
Public Interest
1757 S Street NW
Washington, D.C. 20009
(202) 332-9110

The National Women's Health
Network
224 Seventh Street NE
Washington, D.C. 20003
(202) 543-9222

Cosmetics

Cosmetics, Toiletries and
Fragrance Association
1133 Fifteenth Street NW
Washington, D.C. 20006
(202) 331-1770

Environmental and Occupational Hazards

Environmental Defense Fund
1525 Eighteenth Street NW
Washington, D.C.
(202) 387-3000

Environmental Protection Agency
Waterside Mall, West Tower
401 M Street SW
Washington, D.C. 20460
(202) 382-2090

Laboratory of Reproductive and
Developmental Toxicology
National Institute of Environmental
Health Sciences
P.O. Box 12233
Research Triangle Park, N.C.
27709
(919) 541-2111

National Insitute for Occupational
Safety and Health
5600 Fishers Lane
Rockville, Md. 20857
4676 Columbia Parkway
Cincinnati, Ohio 45226
(513) 684-2876

Women's Occupational Health
Resources Center
Columbia University, School of
Public Health
Room B-106
60 Haven Avenue
New York, N.Y. 10032

NOTE: Many labor unions are also
active in lobbying for safety in the
workplace and can provide
information about specific hazards
in specific industries.

Family Planning

Planned Parenthood Federation of
America
2010 Massachusetts Avenue NW
Washington, D.C. 20036
(202) 785-3351

NOTE: Planned Parenthood
maintains local chapters in most
major cities. These chapters
provide a variety of services
related to family planning. Consult
your telephone directory for local
listings.

Genetic Disorders

Cystic Fibrosis Foundation
3379 Peachtree Road NE
Atlanta, Ga. 30326
(404) 262-1100

Dysautonomia Foundation
370 Lexington Avenue
New York, N.Y. 10017
(212) 889-0300

The March of Dimes Birth Defects
    Foundation
1275 Mamaroneck Avenue
White Plains, N.Y. 10605
(914) 428-7100

National Foundation for Jewish
    Genetic Diseases
608 Fifth Avenue
New York, N.Y. 10020
(212) 541-6340

National Genetics Foundation
555 West 57th Street
New York, N.Y. 10019
(212) 586-5800

National Hemophilia Foundation
25 West 39th Street
New York, N.Y. 10018
(212) 869-9740

National Tay-Sachs and Allied
    Diseases Association
122 East 42nd Street
New York, N.Y. 10017
(212) 661-2780

Sickle Cell Disease Foundation of
    Greater New York
209 West 125th Street
New York, N.Y. 10027
(212) 865-1201

Genetic Disorders
(Counseling Services)

Some of the organizations listed
above provide counseling services.
In addition, a list of counseling
centers throughout the United
States is available, free, from:

The National Center for Education
    in Maternal and Child Health
3520 Prospect Street NW
Washington, D.C. 20057
(202) 625-8400

Health Conditions (Chronic)
That May Affect Pregnancy

American Diabetes Association
2 Park Avenue
New York, N.Y. 10016
(212) 683-7444

American Heart Association
205 East 42nd Street
New York, N.Y. 10017
(212) 661-5335

Epilepsy Foundation of America
4351 Garden City Drive
Landover, Md.
(301) 459-3700

National Kidney Foundation
2 Park Avenue
New York, N.Y. 10016
(212) 683-8018

Health Conditions (Infectious) That May Affect Pregnancy

American Social Health
 Association
260 Sheridan Avenue
Suite 307
Palo Alto, Calif. 94306
VD HOTLINE: Nationwide (800)
 227-8922
 California
 (800) 982-5833

Centers for Disease Control
1600 Clifton Road NE
Atlanta, Ga. 30333
(404) 329-3286

Infertility

American Fertility Society
1608 Thirteenth Avenue
Suite 101
Birmingham, Ala.
(205) 933-7222

Resolve
Box 474
Belmont, Mass. 02178
(617) 484-2424

Midwives (Certified)

The American College of Nurse
 Midwives
1522 K Street NW
Suite 1120
Washington, D.C. 20005
(202) 347-5445

Neonatal Intensive Care

A complete directory of American
hospitals with neonatal intensive
care units (*1982 Guide to Centers
Providing Perinatal and Neonatal
Special Care*) is available at a cost
of $5.00 per copy from:

Ross Planning Associates
Ross Laboratories
Columbus, Ohio 43216
(614) 438-6000

Nutrition

American Dietetic Association
430 North Michigan Avenue
Chicago, Ill. 60611
(312) 822-0330

Food and Nutrition Board
National Academy of Sciences
2101 Constitution Avenue NW
Washington, D.C. 20418
(202) 334-2000

NOTE: Nutrition information is also
available from many other
organizations and agencies listed
here, including The March of
Dimes and The National Center for
Education in Maternal and Child
Health.

Prenatal Care

American College of Obstetricians
 and Gynecologists
One East Wacker Drive
Chicago, Ill. 60601
(312) 222-1600

American Dental Association
212 East Chicago Avenue
Chicago, Ill. 60611
(312) 444-2500

American Foundations for
  Maternal and Child Health
30 Beekman Place
New York, N.Y. 10022
(212) 759-5510

American Medical Association
535 North Dearborn Street
Chicago, Ill. 60610
(312) 751-6000

The National Center for Education
  in Maternal and Child Health
3520 Prospect Street NW
Washington, D.C. 20057
(202) 625-8400

Radiation

National Council on Radiation
  Protection and Measurements
7910 Woodmont Avenue
Bethesda, Md.
(301) 657-2652

U.S. Department of Health and
  Human Services
Bureau of Radiological Health
12720 Twinbrook Parkway HFX1
Rockville, Md. 20852
(301) 443-4690

Sources

PART I **Personal Health**

---

1. How Old Are You?

2. How Much Do You Weigh?
Lauresen, Neils, M.D.; Whitney, Steven, *It's Your Body* (Grosset & Dunlap, 1977).
The Merck Manual, 14th ed. (Merck, Sharp & Dohme, 1982).
Naeye, Richard L., and Tafari, Nebiat, *Risk Factors in Pregnancy and Diseases of the Fetus and Newborn* (Williams & Wilkins, 1983).
"Older moms are nothing new," *Science News,* June 30, 1984.
"Older moms' fetuses may not get enough blood," *Medical World News,* March 28, 1983.
"Sperm change little with age," *Science News,* June 30, 1984.
"Weight loss corrects polycystic ovarian disease in obese women," *Medical World News,* August 22, 1983.

3. Do You Have an Infection?

4. Do You Have a Chronic Condition or Long-Term Disability?
"Active bowel disease a pregnancy risk," *Medical World News,* November 22, 1982.
AMA Drug Evaluations, 5th Ed. (American Medical Association, 1983).
"Aspartame critics persist, recommend avoidance during pregnancy," *Medical World News,* February 27, 1984.
"Herpes virus suspect in nearly a third of miscarriages," *Science News,* June 30, 1984.
The Merck Manual, 14th ed. (Merck, Sharp & Dohme, 1982).
"New crop of PKU victims: babies of successfully treated girls," *Medical World News,* November 23, 1981.
Shepard, Thomas H., *Catalog of Teratogenic Agents,* 4th ed. (Johns Hopkins University Press, 1983).
Spock, Benjamin, *Baby and Child Care* (Pocket Books, 1976).

5. Do You Exercise?
"The Fitness Report," *American Health,* November/December 1983.
"Hot tub use during pregnancy," *Science News,* January 17, 1981.
"Now, the Pregnancy Workout," *Newsweek,* July 23, 1984.

Shepard, Thomas H., *Catalog of Teratogenic Agents*, 4th ed. (Johns Hopkins University Press, 1983).

Slade, Margot, "Keeping fit prudently during pregnancy," *New York Times*, August 6, 1983.

6. Are You Under Emotional Stress?

Kotulak, Ronald, "Your attitude can affect your pregnancy," *Daily News* (N.Y.), February 26, 1980.

Mazor, Miriam D., "The problem of infertility," *The Woman Patient* (Plenum Press, 1978).

U.S. Institute of Medicine, *Research on Stress and Human Health* (National Technical Information Service, 1981).

7. Do You Smoke?

Chemical Hazards to Human Reproduction (Council on Environmental Quality, January 1981).

"Don't smoke while baby is eating," *Science News*, December 6, 1980.

Gilman, Alfred Goodman; Goodman, Louis S.; Gilman, Alfred, eds., *The Pharmacological Basis of Therapeutics*, 6th ed. (Macmillan, 1980).

Rahwan, Ralf G., "Mechanisms of teratogenesis," *U.S. Pharmacist*, March 1983.

"Father's smoking may harm fetuses," Science Watch, *New York Times*, January 18, 1983.

Shepard, Thomas H., *Catalog of Teratogenic Agents*, 4th ed. (Johns Hopkins University Press, 1983).

"Smoking and sperm," *Science News*, April 18, 1981.

"When mom smokes, umbilical cells shrivel," *Medical World News*, January 5, 1981.

PART II **Sex**

---

8. What Kind of Contraception Do You Use?

AMA Drug Evaluations, 5th ed. (American Medical Association, 1983).

Gilman, Alfred Goodman; Goodman, Louis S.; Gilman, Alfred, *The Pharmacological Basis of Therapeutics*, 6th ed. (Macmillan, 1980).

Gossel, Thomas A., "Spermicides: are they safe and effective," *U.S. Pharmacist*, February 1983.

"IUDs and pelvic inflammatory disease," *Science News*, August 20, 1983.

Jick, Hershel, *et al.*, "Vaginal spermicides and congenital disorders," *Journal of the American Medical Association*, April 3, 1981.

"Miscarriage risk tied to intrauterine device," *New York Times*, December 5, 1981.

"PID risk increased sharply among IUD users, British cohort, U.S. case-control studies affirm," *Family Planning Perspectives*, July–August 1981.

Seaman, Barbara; Seaman, Gideon, *Women and the Crisis in Sex Hormones* (Bantam Books, 1979).

Shepard, Thomas H., *Catalog of Teratogenic Agents,* 4th ed. (Johns Hopkins University Press, 1983).

"Spermicide effect on unborn in question," *Science News,* May 15, 1982.

9. **When and How Often Do You Make Love?**

Carrera, Michael, "Sex positions—can they affect your fertility?" *Glamour,* August 1983.

"Intercourse endangers fetus," *Research/Penn State* (Health and Life Sciences), August 1980.

The Merck Manual, 14th ed. (Merck, Sharp & Dohme, 1982).

Naeye, R. L., and Ross, S. M., "Amniotic fluid infection syndrome," *Clinics in Obstetrics and Gynecology,* December 1982.

"Sex during pregnancy," *Glamour,* January 1983.

Shepard, Thomas H., *Catalog of Teratogenic Agents,* 4th ed. (Johns Hopkins University Press, 1983).

PART III **Drugs**

---

10. **Do You Use Illicit Drugs?**

Council on Environmental Quality, *Chemical Hazards to Human Reproduction* (National Technical Information Services, January 1981).

"A fetus can be harmed if Mom smokes pot in pregnancy," *Medical World News,* October 25, 1982.

Gilman, Alfred Goodman; Goodman, Louis S.; Gilman, Alfred, *The Pharmacological Basis of Therapeutics,* 6th Ed. (Macmillan, 1980).

Jacobson, Cecil B.; Berlin, Cheston M., "Possible reproductive detriment in LSD users," *Journal of the American Medical Association,* December 11, 1972.

U.S. Institute of Medicine, *Marijuana and Health* (National Technical Information Service, 1982).

"Marijuana and the reproductive cycle," *Science News,* March 26, 1983.

Martin, Eric, *Hazards of Medication* (Lippincott, 1978).

Nahas, Gabriel G., "When friends or patients ask about . . . marihuana," *Journal of the American Medical Association,* July 7, 1975.

Shepard, Thomas H., *Catalog of Teratogenic Agents,* 4th ed. (Johns Hopkins University Press, 1983).

"THC libido: a little dab will do you," *Science News,* August 15, 1981.

11. **Are You Taking Medication?**

AMA Drug Evaluations, 5th ed. (Americal Medical Association, 1983).

"Assessing childbirth drugs," *FDA Consumer* (U.S., Department of Health, Education and Welfare) December 1979–January 1980.

Berlin, Cheston M., Jr., "Pharmacologic considerations of drug use in lactating mother," *Obstetrics & Gynecology* (supplement), November 1981.

Collins, Edith, "Maternal and fetal effects of acetaminophen and salicylates in pregnancy," *Obstetrics & Gynecology* (supplement), November 1981.

"Drug information forum," *U.S. Pharmacist,* October 1981.

Gilman, Alfred Goodman; Goodman, Louis S.; Gilman, Alfred, *The Pharmacological Basis of Therapeutics,* 6th ed. (Macmillan, 1980).

The Merck Manual, 14th ed. (Merck, Sharp & Dohme, 1982).

Miller, Donald R.; Tanner N. Steven, "Thromboembolism during pregnancy and lactation," *U.S. Pharmacist,* May 1983.

The Physicians' Desk Reference, 36th ed. (Medical Economics Company, 1982).

Poirer, Theresa I., "Factors involved in adverse drug reactions," *U.S. Pharmacist,* April 1983.

Randal, Judith, "Acne drug linked to other illness," *Daily News* (N.Y.), September, 11, 1983.

Rudolf, Abraham M., "The effects of nonsteroidal antiinflammatory compounds on fetal circulation and pulmonary function," *Obstetrics & Gynecology* (supplement), November 1981.

Schwarz, Richard H., "Consideration of antibiotic therapy during pregnancy," *Obstetrics & Gynecology* (supplement), November 1981.

Shepard, Thomas H., *Catalog of Teratogenic Agents,* 4th ed. (John Hopkins University Press, 1983).

Shnider, Sol M., "Choice of anesthesia for labor and delivery," *Obstetrics & Gynecology* (supplement), November 1981.

Witter, Frank R., et al., "The effects of chronic gastrointestinal medication on the fetus and neonate," *Obstetrics & Gynecology* (supplement), November 1981.

"Valium, cleft palate untied," *Science News,* December 13, 1983.

"Valproic acid increases risks of birth defects," *Medical World News,* December 6, 1982.

Vorherr, Helmuth, et al., "Vaginal adsorption of povidone-iodine," *Journal of the American Medical Association,* December 1980.

PART IV Medical Procedures

12. Do You Need an Immunization?

AMA Drug Evaluations, 5th ed. (American Medical Association, 1983).

"Fetus vaccinations reported," *New York Times,* September 11, 1983.

The Merck Manual, 14th ed. (Merck, Sharp & Dohme, 1982.

Centers for Disease Control, *Morbidity and Mortality Weekly Report,*

November 2, 1979,; February 22, 1980; February 29, 1980; February 6, 1981; June 19, 1981.

13. Has Your Doctor Suggested X-Rays?

Effects of Ionizing Radiation on Developing Embryo and Fetus: A Review (U.S. Dept. of Health and Human Services, Bureau of Radiological Health), August 1981.

NCRP Report No. 54: Medical Radiation Exposure of Pregnant and Potentially Pregnant Women (National Council on Radiation Protection and Measurement, September 15, 1979).

Procedures to Minimize Diagnostic X-Ray Exposure of the Human Embryo and Fetus (U.S. Department of Health and Human Services, Bureau of Radiological Health, August 1981).

"Radiation and birth defects," *March of Dimes Science News Information File,* August 1979.

14. Have You Had an Abortion?

"Abortion doesn't lower fertility," *Medical World News,* December 20, 1982.

Multiple Induced Abortions May Harm Later Childbearing (March of Dimes Birth Defects Foundation, June 23, 1980).

Shepard, Thomas H., *Catalog of Teratogenic Agents,* 4th ed. (Johns Hopkins University Press, 1983).

15. Where Will You Have Your Baby?

National Institutes of Health, *Cesarean Childbirth,* Consensus Development Conference Summary, Vol. 3, No. 6, 1980.

"Debate over preoperative shaving leaves surgeons splitting hairs," *Medical World News,* October 10, 1983.

Goodell, Rae; Gurin, Joel, "Where should babies be born?" *American Health,* January/February 1984.

The Merck Manual, 14th ed. (Merck, Sharp & Dohme, 1982).

Boston Women's Health Collective, *Our Bodies, Ourselves* (Simon & Schuster, 1979).

Rosenthal, Diane J., "Choices in Childbirth," *Rx Being Well,* May/June 1983.

"Silastic cup deliveries outscore use of forceps for maternal safety," *Medical World News,* March 12, 1984.

PART V **Nutrition**

---

16. What Do You Eat and Drink?

"A Look at diet regimes," *U.S. Pharmacist,* August 1982.

Alternative Dietary Practices and Nutritional Abuses in Pregnancy (National Research Council, 1982).

AMA Drug Evaluations, 5th ed. (American Medical Association, 1983).

Beller, Anne Scott, *Fat and Thin* (Farrar, Straus & Giroux, 1977).

Claire M. Cassidy, "Subcultural prenatal diets of Americans," *Alter-*

native Dietary Practices and Nutritional Abuses in Pregnancy (National Research Council, 1982).

Dairy Council Digest (National Dairy Council), January–February 1979.

"Danger of lead in canned foods," *New York Times,* April 2, 1983, and "Lead Soldering Warning,' *New York Times,* December 8, 1982.

Dwyer, Johanna, "Vegetarian diets in pregnancy," *Alternative Dietary Practices and Nutritional Abuses in Pregnancy* (National Research Council, 1982).

Farb, Peter; Armelagos, George, *Consuming Passions: The Anthropology of Eating* (Houghton Mifflin, 1980).

Fetal Alcohol Syndrome Linked to Zinc Deficiency (Vanderbilt University Medical Center, November 1982).

Frisch, R.; MacArthur, J., "Menstrual cycles: fatness as a determinant of minimum weight for height necessary for their maintainance or onset," *Science,* vol. 185 (1974), quoted in Anne Scott Beller, *Fat and Thin* (Farrar, Straus & Giroux, 1977).

Gilman, Alfred Goodman; Goodman, Louis S.; Gilman, Alfred, *The Pharmacological Basis of Therapeutics,* 6th ed. (Macmillan, 1980).

Grishan, Fayez K.; Greene, Harry L., "Fetal alcohol syndrome: failure of zinc supplementation to reverse the effect of ethanol on placental transport of zinc," *Pediatric Research,* July 1983.

Jacobson, Michael, *Eater's Digest* (Anchor Books, 1976).

Linn, Shai, *et al.,* "No association between coffee consumption and adverse outcomes of pregnancy," *New England Journal of Medicine,* January 21, 1982.

The March of Dimes, press release, August 1979.

Martin, Eric, *Hazards of Medication* (Lippincott, 1978).

The Merck Manual, 14th ed. (Merck, Sharp & Dohme, 1982).

Metzger, Boyd E.; Vileisis, Rita A.; Ravnikar, Veronica; Fredinkel, Norbert, " 'Accelerated starvation' and the skipped breakfast in late normal pregnancy," *The Lancet,* March 13, 1982.

New York State Department of Health, news releases, August 5, 1981, October 15, 1982.

Recommended Dietary Allowances (National Research Council, 1980).

Rosenberg, Lynn, *et al.,* "Selected birth defects in relation to caffeine-containing beverages," *Journal of the American Medical Association,* March 12, 1982.

Rosett, Henry L., *et al.,* "Patterns of alcohol consumption and fetal development," *Obstetrics & Gynecology,* May 1983.

Seaman, Barbara; Seaman, Gideon, *Women and the Crisis in Sex Hormones* (Bantam Books, 1979).

"Sexual development and teen drinking," *Science News,* May 2, 1981.

Shepard, Thomas H., *Catalog of Teratogenic Agents,* 4th ed. (Johns Hopkins University Press, 1983).

17. Are There Harmful Additives in Your Food?

Freydberg, Nicholas; Gortner, Willis, *The Food Additives Book* (Bantam, 1982).

Jacobson, Michael F., *Eater's Digest* (Anchor Books, 1976).

Registry of Toxic Effects of Chemical Substances (National Institute for Occupational Safety and Health, 1982).

Shepard, Thomas H., *Catalog of Teratogenic Agents,* 4th ed. (Johns Hopkins University Press, 1983).

Winter, Ruth, *A Consumer's Dictionary of Food Additives* (Crown, 1978).

18. Do You Take Vitamin and Mineral Supplements?

Bernhardt, Irwin B.; Darsey, James D., "Hypervitaminosis A and congenital renal anomalies," *Obstetrics & Gynecology,* May 974.

"Chemistry," *Science News,* January 21, 1983.

Cochrane, W. A., "Overnutrition in prenatal and neonatal life a problem?," *Journal of the Canadian Medical Association,* October 23, 1965.

Copper Stimulates a Hormone Essential to Ovulation (University of Texas Health Science Center at Dallas, June 14, 1962).

Dwyer, Johanna; "Vegetarian diets in pregnancy," *Alternative Dietary Practices and Nutritional Abuses in Pregnancy* (National Research Council, 1982).

Edelson, Edward, "Link a major birth defect to poor food habits," *Daily News* (N.Y.), December 27, 1980.

"Fluoride compounds," *Accepted Dental Therapeutics* (American Dental Association, 1982).

Graedon, Joe, *The People's Pharmacy* (St. Martin's Press, 1976).

"Infertile women conceive after vitamin B_6 therapy," *Medical World News,* March 19, 1979.

Interview with Dr. Pedro Rosso, Columbia Institute on Human Nutrition, 1980.

Low Sperm Counts Linked to Zinc Deficiency, American Chemical Society News Service, March 29, 1982.

Gilman, Alfred Goodman; Goodman, Louis S.; Gilman, Alfred, *The Pharmacological Basis of Therapeutics,* 6th ed. (Macmillan, 1980).

Martin, Eric, *Hazards of Medication* (Lippincott, 1978).

Meadows, N. J., *et al.,* "Zinc and small babies," *The Lancet,* November 21, 1981.

The Merck Manual, 14th ed., (Merck, Sharp & Dohme, 1982).

Milk-Based and Soy-Based Formulations Used for Feeding Term Infants at Home" (Ross Laboratories, June 1982).

Recommended Dietary Allowances (National Research Council, 1980).

"Science Puts Pressure on Calcium," *American Health,* January/February, 1984.

Shepard, Thomas H., *Catalog of Teratogenic Agents,* 4th ed. (Johns Hopkins University Press, 1983).

Smithells, R. W., *et al.,* "Possible prevention of neural-tube defects by periconceptional vitamin supplementation," *The Lancet,* February 16, 1980.

"Vitamin and mineral drug products for over-the-counter human use," *Federal Register,* March 16, 1979, Part II.

PART VI The Environment

19. Where Do You Work?

Chavkin, W.; Welch, L., *Occupational Hazards to Reproduction* (The Program in Occupational Health and The Residency Program in Social Medicine, Montefiore Hospital and Medical Center [N.Y.], 1980).

Council on Environmental Quality, *Chemical Hazards to Human Reproduction* (National Technical Information Service, January 1981).

"EtO dangers prompt new standard," *Science News,* January 22, 1983.

Garmon, Lisa, "Puzzled over PCBs," *Science News,* May 29, 1982.

Gilman, Alfred Goodman; Goodman, Louis S.; Gilman, Alfred, *The Pharmacological Basis of Therapeutics,* 6th ed. (Macmillan, 1980).

"Lead absorption may provide clue to sudden infant death syndrome," *Medical World News,* October 10, 1983.

Hamilton, Cindy W., "Risk to personnel admixing cancer chemotherapy," *U.S. Pharmacist,* July 1982.

Martin, Eric, *Hazards of Medication* (Lippincott, 1978).

"Occupational exposure to high heat linked to subsequent male infertility," *Medical World News,* July 9, 1984.

"Pesticides: the human body burden," *Science News,* September 24, 1983.

Pregnancy and VDT Workers: Pressure Leads to a Quest for Hard Facts," *Business Week,* April 23, 1984.

Rahwan, Ralf, "Mechanisms of Teratogenesis," *U.S. Pharmacist,* March 1983.

Rawls, Rebecca, "Reproductive hazards in the workplace," *Chemical Engineering News,* February 11, 1980.

Registry of Toxic Effects of Chemical Substance (National Institute for Occupational Safety and Health, February 1982).

Schmeck, Harold M., Jr., "Study finds use of 'laughing gas' may be hazard to dental workers," *New York Times,* October 15, 1979.

Shepard, Thomas H., *Catalog of Teratogenic Agents,* 4th ed. (Johns Hopkins University Press, 1983).

Thomas, John A., "Reproductive hazards and environmental chemicals: a review," *Toxic Substances Journal,* Vol. 2, No. 4, 1981.

20. How Safe Is Your Home?

Blumenthal, Deborah, "The problems of pregnancy," *New York Times Magazine,* Feburary 13, 1983.

Chavkin, W.; Welch, L., *Occupational Hazards to Reproduction* (The Program in Occupational Health and the Residency Program in Social Medicine, Montefiore Hospital and Medical Center [N.Y.], 1980).

Council on Environmental Quality, *Chemical Hazards to Human Reproduction* (National Technical Information Service, January 1981).

Gosselin, Robert E.; Hodge, Harold C.; Smith, Roger P.; Gleason, Marion N., *Clinical Toxicology of Commercial Products,* 4th ed. (Williams & Wilkins, 1976).

"The health effects of cooking with gas," *Science News,* October 24, 1981.

"Study finds pollutants emitted by gas heaters," *New York Times,* August 4, 1983.

Zamm, Alfred V., with Gannon, Robert, *Why Your Home May Endanger Your Health* (Simon & Schuster, 1980).

21. Do You Plan to Travel?

The Merck Manual, 14th ed. (Merck, Sharp & Dohme, 1982).

NCRP Report #45: Natural Background Radiation in the United States (National Council on Radiation Protection, November 1975).

NCRP Report #54: Medical Radiation Exposure of Pregnant and Potentially Pregnant Women (National Council on Radiation Protection, September 15, 1979).

Rubovits, Frank E., "Traumatic rupture of the pregnant uterus from 'seat belt' injury," *American Journal of Obstetrics and Gynecology,* November 15, 1964.

PART VII **Tests You Should Know About**

A Listing of Genetic Diseases for Which Diagnostic Tests Are Available Through the Genetic Counseling and Treatment Network (National Genetics Foundation, 1972).

"Antibody tests promise better diagnosis of herpes simplex infection . . ." and ". . . plus two other sexually transmitted diseases," *Medical World News,* March 14, 1983.

Boffey, Philip M., " 'Safe' form of radiation arouses new worry," *New York Times,* August 2, 1983.

"Drug information forum," *U.S. Pharmacist,* September 1982.

"FDA approves alpha-fetoprotein kit amid physician, consumer concerns," *Medical World News,* July 15, 1983.

"Help is coming for herpes," *Time,* June 27, 1983.

"Hamster egg assay validated," *Medical World News,* May 23, 1983.

"Is she or isn't she pregnant? How they found out in King Tut's time," press release on pregnancy testing kits prepared by Ruder & Finn, Inc., New York, October 27, 1978.

The Merck Manual, 14th ed. (Merck, Sharp & Dohme, 1982).

Minutes of the meeting of the clinical chemistry section of the clinical chemistry and hematology devices panel (professional adviser to the Food and Drug Administration Bureau of Medical Devices), December 4, 1978.

"New test for birth defects," *Science News,* August 20, 1983.

Pinckney, Cathey; Pinckney, Edward, *The Patient's Guide to Medical Tests* (Facts on File, 1982).

Powledge, Tabitha M., "Windows on the world," *Psychology Today,* May 1983.

"Prenatal diagnosis of genetic disease," *Modern Medicine/OB-GYN Guide* (reprint), (National Genetics Foundation, 1978).

Schmeck, Harold M., Jr., "New prenatal test raises concern for fetus," *New York Times,* May 27, 1984.

"Speedy OTC pregnancy test combines at-home simplicity, lab precision," *Medical World News,* August 22, 1983.

Stedman's Medical Dictionary, 24th ed. (Williams & Wilkins, 1982).

Stephenson, Sharon R.; Weaver, David D., "Prenatal diagnosis—a compilation of diagnosed conditions," *American Journal of Obstetrics and Gynecology,* October, 1981.

Should You Consider Amniocentesis? (The National Genetics Foundation, n.d.).

Index

℗

Related Titles from PLUME

(0452)